The Light Touch

An Easy Guide to Hands-On-Healing

The Light Touch

An Easy Guide to Hands-On-Healing

Judie Chiappone, RN, LMT

THE LIGHT TOUCH. Copyright © 1987 by Judie Chiappone.
Revised in 1989. Revised Expanded Edition in 2001.

All rights reserved, including the right to reproduce this book or portions thereof in any form whatsoever — without written permission from the author. For more information write:

Judie Chiappone
183 Largo Drive
Poinciana, Florida 34759
Email: Judie@SacredChoices.com
Web site: www.SacredChoices.com

Cover Illustration by Tina Meck
Production and typography by Cathy Sanders

The techniques and philosophies in this book are not meant to be used for diagnosing or prescribing, nor are they meant to be used in place of sound medical care. In the event that you use any information in this book for yourself or others, the author assumes no responsibility for your actions.

To Carl and Lincoln

Table of Contents

Chapter 1 The Gift Of Intimidation! 17

Chapter 2 Will The Real Healer Please Rise! 21

Chapter 3 What "It" Is...What "It" Does! 27

Chapter 4 Reality...On An Energy Level! 33

Chapter 5 Getting Started 37
  - The Connection...A Balancing Act 39
  - Remaining On Center While Healing 40

Chapter 6 Six Steps In Healing 41
  - The Triple Awareness Breath 41
  - The Scan 41
  - Unruffling...The Fun Step! 44
  - Intervention Techniques 46
  - Grounding The Healee 49
  - Terminating The Treatment 50

Chapter 7 Specific Intervention Techniques 53
  - The Energy Flow 53
  - Unruffling 53

- Massage 54
- Double Hand Boost 55
- Laser 56
- Ultrasound 57
- The Siphon 58
- Fluffing The Aura 60
- Reflexology...The Painless Way! 61
- The Back Package 62
  - –Massage 62
  - –The Thumb Walk 62
  - –The Hopi Indian Technique 64
  - –Ultrasound 69
- Boosting And Balancing The Chakras 69
- The Buddy System 73
- The "Magnificent 7" 74
- Full Balancing Of Major And Minor Chakras 75

Chapter 8   Three Approaches To Healing 79

Chapter 9   The Tiny Clients...Infants! 81
- The Touch Itself...What Was That You Said? 82
- Anne And Jeffery...A Tiny Love Story 83

Chapter 10   Healing Enhancers 87
- The Importance of Intention 87
- Detaching Yourself From Outcomes 87
- Visualization 88
- Simplifying 89
- Unconditional Love 90
- Expecting 92
- Energy Pillows 92

Chapter 11 **A Quick Reference For Specific Problems** 95

Chapter 12 **Delightful Demos**..97
- Post-Operative 97
- Strokes..99
- Eye Injuries..100
- Cancer 101
- Angina 102
- Premature Infants..103
- Broken Bones...104
- Sunburn...104
- Plants 105
- Animals 105

Chapter 13 **Living In Healing Ways**..................................107
- Self-Talk = Cell Talk!..108
- Gentle Care And Feeding Of The Psychological You!...113
- Gentle Care And Feeding Of The Emotional You!........114
- Your Back Speaks 116
- You're Excited About Healing, You Want To Share It...But How? 117
- Delegating Responsibility..119
- Healing In The Workplace 120
- Nurses 121
- Massage Therapists 122
- Distance Healing 122
- More Ideas For Living In Healing Ways......................123

Suggested Resources...127

Introduction

As an admiring friend and grateful client, I requested the privilege of writing the introduction to this joyful little book. Then I panicked! How does one tie a ribbon 'round a rainbow? Or capture a sunbeam in the cup of one's hands? How do you lasso laughter? Especially, how does one adequately elucidate unconditional love?

The best way I know is to "tell it like it was."

Judie Chiappone, more appropriately pronounced Judie "Cheerupa," R.N., Nurse Practitioner, Instructor in "Therapeutic Touch," Licensed Massage Therapist, and author, came into my life as a true "ball of lightening." (Yes, that's the way I meant to spell it!) Light, laughter, and love are Judie's constant traveling companions, along with the rainbow she leaves behind when she departs.

When Judie, with those great blue eyes set in a luminous smile, comes floating through your doorway, deftly maneuvering that huge folding massage table, you know from the radiance that accompanies her that *something* is going to happen. I can tell you from experience that something *wonderful* does!

Judie appeared on my horizon at a time when my morale was lying on its back trying with both hands and both feet to prevent the sky, which had fallen on me, from smothering me.

This (then 75 year old) charter member of the "lunatic fringe" (those who take responsibility for their own health by learning and attempting to put into practice the "New Age" techniques such as natural food diets, exercise, positive mental attitudes, etc., for staying healthy, happy and productive for a long time) was suffering from an acute and critical case of "Why me?" Suffice it to say that every aspect of my life was thrown suddenly into a state of flux. Tho' I did not "fit the profile" in ANY way, I had been informed that I must undergo major surgery for the "BIG ONE." Consequently, because I could no longer care for her, I would lose the congenial companionship of my ailing friend/business partner/housemate of many years. This possibly meant selling our lovely home and my finding another place to live. And, as though all this were not enough, current problems in the business we'd spent more than 25 years building had caused the termination of a substantial part of our income on which we had counted for security in our declining years. (So how was your day?)

It was into this disaster area that Judie dropped from what sky remained up there, accompanied by her own very special brand of what I call her "Triple L-T"...light, laughter, love, and touch administered to the celestial strains of harp solos on her portable stereo.

Funny thing. Often you don't even *feel* the touch! But the light, the laughter, and the love she radiates the moment she walks into a room, and all the while she works, begin to flow gently through your body (*and* your mind *and* your spirit) in soft soothing waves of healing like the gentle vibrations of the music from the harp. You close your eyes and begin to allow yourself to relax and just to "be." Judie's sensitive hands waft above your body, sensing and unscrambling any energy blockages she intuitively encounters in your being.

She may or may not offer comments, depending upon what

your body tells her about you. The first time Judie treated me in late 1986, she concluded the hour with a startling statement. It seems my body had told her "that I did not have a blockage. *My whole left side was a solid granite wall!*" She told me gently that, "you must start loving yourself, and begin to pour the same wonderful love into yourself that you so freely give to everyone around you. Your family (including those forty-five nieces and nephews) and a multitude of friends know very well of your unconditional love and unending support for them. You need to put yourself at the top of that list... and treat yourself just as you would the most precious friend you have! Your body is screaming with this message. Listen to it! Love it! Disease is merely our body's way of getting us to do for ourselves what we've refused to do in the past. Love is its basic nature. It can't do without it and remain silent! The longer the neglect, the stronger the message will be. Health is NOT just perfection in nutrition, positive attitudes, and exercise. Ongoing nurturing with self-love is the catalyst for health."

Love myself! Indeed!

I'd been raised to believe that "to love one's self is vain and that vanity is a sin! I'd never had any trouble avoiding that sin! All I had to do was look in the mirror! How could anybody love what I saw there? Big nose, crooked teeth, poker straight red hair... and if the mirror chanced to be full length, there staring stolidly back at me was the five foot seven inch round-shouldered, gangling, awkward creature I'd repeatedly been told I was since I was twelve. Now, at 75, the freckles had faded, and euphemistically "the gold had turned to silver" and the shoulders grown rounder still.

Love myself!

But Judie had managed to get my attention. Especially when shortly thereafter a second opinion confirmed the dreaded "diagnosis."

Two days after Judie's first visit, the mail brought from her a tape filled with "love myself" songs, messages, and techniques along with an assignment. First thing I was to do every morning when I got up was to look in the mirror and say out loud "I love you!" Now that took some doing from this old crow! But I'm doing it! (First I say, "Good morning God, I love you!")

Someone once said, "Life is what happens when you are making other plans." What happened to me was not what I had planned at all! Why did it take so long for me to learn the REAL facts of life?

On a dreary rainy Sunday afternoon in January, the day before I was to enter the hospital, Judie appeared at my door on her way to a social occasion. Her trusty table in hand, complete with an electric sheet to keep me warm, she had come to give me a "treatment" as a preparation for my surgery.

She also brought me a present. A small 6x6x1 inch cotton flannel pillow stuffed with raw bale cotton. Judie had "energized" it by merely holding it in her hands and allowing energy from the cosmos to flow into it. She explained that if I kept the pillow close to my incision it could minimize any pain I might have. I accepted her gift with faith and much gratitude.

"Balancing my energy patterns" was finished in good time for Judie's dinner engagement. And, having filled me to the brim with positive programming, she assured me she'd never worked on a patient better primed for successful surgery. Before leaving, she promised to come to the hospital to "balance me" again after surgery.

I received a total of seven treatments from Judie. She peppered me with tapes, cards, and phone calls, continually reminding me to look in the mirror and say, "I love you!" (By now, I'm actually beginning to like the old gal I see there. She's really a very nice person!) My surgery was on Tuesday afternoon. The following Friday at noon, having done my own packing up, I walked out of my hospital room to go home. Behind me, I left three shifts of gracious nurses and a slightly incredulous surgeon who kept offering prescriptions for pain, which I steadfastly refused. (I might add in passing that I deliberately delayed my surgery until my biorhythms were in a triple high.)

When Judie first treated me, I expressed concern about my draining her energy. She assured me that she was not using her energy. She was merely acting as a conduit through which "universal energy" was being channeled, and that she was also being energized by the process at the same time.

As instructed, I kept Judie's "energy pillow" close to my long incision and have neither required nor taken ANY drugs in any form at any time then or since. With the exception of one bout with the flu in March 1988 (which I weathered without drugs also), I have not spent a full day in bed since I left the hospital. It is now two years and seven months since my surgery. In summary, these are the facts:

- Believing as I do, that my body is my property, and that therefore I am responsible for it... and should have the freedom to choose how I permit it to be treated, I chose to decline all the various "killer" therapies which are the usual protocol following the surgery I had.

- Instead, I researched in detail and adopted several alternative therapies designed to detoxify the body and to fortify the immune system by regenerating the body at the cellular level.

- I have come to believe that my body is an integral part of an intricate and magnificent Universe that is governed by definite laws ordained by its Creator. If I observe as assiduously as I can the laws for nurturing and preserving my body, mind, and spirit, I firmly believe that the God who created me will continue daily to re-create healthy cells in my body.

This has become a learning process I have found illuminating, rewarding, and exhilarating; and I shall continue it for life.

At age 78 now, I am happy and grateful to report that my energy level, my general sense of well-being, and my outlook on life continue on an upward curve.

Since Judie taught me to open the door to loving myself, love has poured through that door in great warming waves from everywhere. Friends and relatives from all over the country rallied with loving support, and continue to stand "at the ready."

Indeed, I've discovered that love is the best medicine there is, and it's the only kind I take!

This, then, is simply a testament to the miracle of healing that can take place in one desolate and despairing life when a "Judie Chiappone" appears, bearing her incalculable gifts of "Light, Love, Laughter and Touch." It is more than that. It is a vignette of true unconditional love in action. It is proof of what can happen to you, no matter how late or how low, when someone *OUT OF AND WITH UNCONDITIONAL LOVE* teaches you how to love yourself, and how to let others love you, too!

Life tossed me a challenge. I'm trying to mold of it a chalice with which to drink more deeply of life.

May you experience this miracle. Better still may you know the joy of giving it away!

God's in heaven (in me!) and all's coming right with my world! Thank you, Judie! Thank you, everyone! Thank you, God! God Bless you with love!

M.C.

Chapter I

The Gift Of Intimidation!

I can remember so many instances in my years of traditional nursing when everything that I knew to do as a nurse just wasn't enough. The maximum dose of pain medication brought little relief...or in other cases, the wound or fracture just wouldn't heal. For dying patients or for their loved ones, words just weren't enough. And, there in the midst of it all were a number of co-workers suffering from obvious stress and burnout. They too were in need of nurturing and healing as they felt the frustrations of not being able to DO something. Well, for myself and thousands of "regular" people (those with no apparent "natural gifts" for healing) healing through touch has been a marvelous answer and one that deeply resounds to the "nurse" or "helper" in so many of us.

Now, you'd think that with all my enthusiasm for this process, that I must have been a real "natural" in this work, huh! Guess again! I had a familiar old cassette playing in my head and it goes something like "Everyone's getting this except me!"

A number of years ago, I was an unsuspecting "regular" person looking for a fun course to take in order to get my continuing education units for my nursing license. I discovered a course called "Therapeutic Touch," which is a healing process made popular by Dr. Dolores Krieger. It stems from the ancient art of laying on of hands. I signed up for the course not knowing that it was about healing. Sounded good to me...I liked the title, liked to "touch," and thought adding a "therapeutic" element was perfect for my role as a nurse!

Well, there came a moment of reckoning in the very first class...we were supposed to share what we had felt in the previous "scanning" exercise (scanning the energy field of our partner with our hands). My mouth dropped open as I listened to fellow classmates excitedly describe all the "differences" they had noted...areas in which they felt heat, static electricity, congestion, and even colors that they saw around their partner! *I HAD FELT NOTHING!* Some even claimed that they were totally dubious of the process, and yet even they were able to experience these unusual findings. I found it all rather intimidating...yet quite inspiring! Who could have guessed that this one course would point me on one of the most important and rewarding paths in my life, that of a "Healing Journey"! And, who could have guessed what a wonderful treasure would emerge from such an intimidating experience!

As the course progressed, we learned a few fundamental healing techniques. I began trying them on a number of friends who had assorted ailments. To my amazement, I began gathering a few "demos," (my term for "outward demonstrations of healing" or, seeing "obvious results"!) The pain in the shoulder disappeared, headaches faded away, cramps disappeared, etc. All of that, as I walked through the process with the intent to help or heal...but felt nothing!

After this beginning class in Therapeutic Touch (TT), I eagerly signed up for Advanced TT, Practitioner TT, and then Instructor. I began blending it in with my work as a Licensed

Massage Therapist. Soon I became quite accustomed to witnessing daily miracles in my life...the latest miracle bringing with it the same fresh delight and ongoing amazement that accompanied the very first one I had witnessed!

I want to set the stage for you...there I was, successfully utilizing TT on a daily basis, teaching it to others, and guess what? I still wasn't able to sense or feel anything on an energy level with my own two hands!

What's my point in all this? Whether you are a "feeler" or a "non-feeler" is not the issue in effectively doing this work. I'm here to tell you that at this very moment...*you are fully equipped and capable* of learning the joy of "hands-on-healing." The key lies in that you lovingly allow yourself to unfold in your own unique style. As you do the exercises, if you happen to sense something as you "listen with your hands"...that's great! If you feel nothing...that's great too! Or perhaps you fall in-between... once in a while you pick up something. Wherever you are at the moment in this business of sensing, I'm here to guide you along the way and to show you just how easy it can be.

What I am sharing with you in this book is merely A way... there are many ways to facilitate healing in others. (There is my way, and your way...there is no *THE* way!) I'm sharing my truth, my philosophy, and what has worked and is working extremely well for me. I now invite you to see what you can "internally validate" as being your own truth, while you enjoy your personal journey in *The Light Touch*.

Chapter 2

Will The Real Healer Please Rise?

(A look at the roles we each play in the healing process...)

Some call me a healer. More accurately I am merely a channel, vehicle, or instrument used to facilitate the well-being (or wholeness) of another...because no one heals another person! The healing is always done by the one receiving. (But then, you knew that!) I merely have the honor of "showing up" and energetically enticing them into wholeness. While most equate healing with "fixing the something that is wrong" or "ridding the body of disease or dysfunction," I see it as a moment of expanding into a greater truth and opening to the flow of Life Force that we've temporarily pinched off. It's about opening to health rather than stomping out disease. As a healer, you might say that I have the honor of energetically reminding others of who they really are! This is an honor I'm never bored with.

No matter how honored and thrilled I am to participate, the person receiving the healing treatment (the "healee") always has the final say and can literally block all healing efforts, or let them in. It is not possible to "assert" healing into anyone's life against their will. So, while I'm playing the role of the healer, the healee is always in charge. This point is one that sometimes has to be learned repeatedly. Your position as a healer (if you care to accept it), is a delightful one in the neutral zone. This is somewhere between the urge to jump up and down yelling, "I did it...I did it!" (the other end of the spectrum) and "I failed!" Both are the old ego talking. The ego has a difficult time remembering who the healer is!

Some of the worst times are when you have a personal stake in the situation. For example, you are treating a loved one and desperately want them to be well. Or, you're out to prove to someone else "that this stuff really works!" Oooh, you failed! Gotcha! I used to handle this by mentally asking my ego to wait in the corner of the room until I was through...but then decided that this wasn't a very loving thing to do to part of my wonderful "self." (I'm very much into daily strides to love myself unconditionally!) Since then, I still have my ego mentally journey to a corner of the room, but I send an imaginary therapist who gives it a loving massage during the wait! Works for me!

One of the easiest ways to clarify the role each of us plays in any healing (our own or others) is to talk about the source of this marvelous healing energy. The energy that I'm speaking of has been utilized by people all over the world since ancient times. Some call it "prana," "bio-cosmic energy," "chi," "life force," etc. (May the "force" be with you!...from the movie *Star Wars*.) Christ called it "light." The latter is my favorite since it seems to visually portray just what I mentally see happening when I place my hands on another person with the intent of healing. Energy, in the form of light, flows from my hands into the person's body, lighting up every little cell in its path...lighting up dark and stagnant areas, and in turn, re-establishing energy flow and balance where there were blocks.

For me this has become a deeply spiritual (as opposed to religious) experience—of tapping into the divine. Whether you call this source God, Christ, Holy Spirit, Buddha, Universe, Universal Mind, etc., it is truly an unlimited source of divine healing energy. The wonderful thing about it is that as it flows from your "source" through you to the healee, you are also the recipient. You benefit by feeling marvelous as well. If instead, you feel depleted and drained, chances are you are using your own energy reserve. (Sooo, may the "Source" be with you!)

The divine aspect of this energy likens it to sending pure, unconditional love. It often seems to me like loving another person into wellness! (Whatever wellness state they're ready for.)

Let's talk for a moment about the "healee" (the one receiving). On a soul level, we all have lessons to learn and paths to walk as we learn. The degree to which a "complete healing" (as opposed to symptomatic relief) can take place is governed in part by a bigger, or you might say, deeper picture. Pain, disease and dysfunction are marvelous ways to get you to pay attention to your very own life! It's important to look at the "a-HA" or the "punch line" associated with any problem. (There is one, you know!) Illness can provide a marvelous opportunity to truly embrace a richness of life itself. Perhaps you've heard the common truth found among those critically ill...that it wasn't until they were dying that they truly began to live!

We're full of excuses for not taking time out for ourselves. Our world is filled with "musts" and "shoulds" and "have to's!" The laundry is piling up at this very moment! Our "inner selves" (souls) have heard that one before! We are all too often just plain "out of balance" in the "giving and receiving" department. Along the way, in the middle of all the "busy"-ness, we create a number of opportunities to return to balance. We experience these moments as short stretches of "down time" or "time outs"...little annoying illnesses which provide a perfect time to nurture ourselves and reflect on life...a perfect time to play the role of the "healee." But, all too often, we merely find the experience frustrating or a nuisance. We trudge onward with life's duties, in spite of the illness, moving a little more slowly, and possibly upset that we're getting farther behind!

If we're lucky, we may even create a health crisis! (Did she say lucky?) One we truly can't ignore. Bingo! We finally got our own attention!

A truly motivated healee can find a whole new world of health linked with modalities such as guided meditation, biofeedback, hands-on-healing, dancing, exercising, visualization, acupuncture, art therapy, singing, massage, nutritional therapy (including supplements), and a host of others.

And, ah yes, we mustn't forget one more modality, which we all need, called laughter! As you laugh, your liver, stomach, spleen, pancreas and other organs all laugh too! They aren't laughing *at* you...they're laughing *with* you, on a cellular level! And at the very same moment, your entire well-being is given a boost...your immune system is absolutely grinning! Can you visualize it? The prescription reads, "You are ordered to have side-splitting, tear-producing, convulsive laughter, four times a day and PRN (short for "as necessary")!" By the way, have you ever noticed how impossible it is to focus on a fear or a worry and laugh uproariously at the same time? Repeat after me... "HEALING IS FUN!" "I CHOOSE LIFE!" (There's nothing like a motivated healee!)

The healing process involves more than just the desire to get well. It involves a leap in the awareness of how life is being processed down deep inside (Where are you holding resentments, or holding back on forgiveness and love?) It is a creative dance that includes new ideas for living in healing ways that promote a sense of balance on a daily basis. A passive "do me, do me" attitude on the part of the healee just doesn't get the job done. Healing needs to be sought through greater personal awareness and participation.

So you see, healing can be enhanced in many ways. The healee can be found in various states of readiness to allow healing on both conscious and unconscious levels, and literally controls the process. This is where you, the healer, come in! You have the joy of connecting one with the other (healee with the healing), along with ideas for the gentle care and feeding of a seeker of health! (No strings attached!)

Chapter 3

What "It" Is...
What "It" Does!

I look at hands-on-healing as "jump starting" the body on a cellular level. The energy is offered, and the cells begin to hum in perfect harmony, enhancing the body's natural ability to self-correct and accelerate healing. This is very similar to the ancient art of laying-on-of-hands but with a new A-HA! It was previously felt that this was only performed as a religious ceremony and by a person chosen by God to channel the healing. It has been demonstrated repeatedly by Dr. Dolores Krieger and hundreds of practitioners, that this is a natural human potential and can be learned by anyone with a sincere desire to participate in the healing process. That's right, even you and me!

Tests done by Dr. Krieger include evidence of increased hemoglobin and hematocrit (oxygen carrying ability of the red blood cells) in patients treated with Therapeutic Touch (TT), while the control group remained unchanged. Other studies included watering plants with specially treated water (ordinary water energized with a healer's hands). Unlike the plants that received the same water but "untreated," these plants had a significant increase in their chlorophyll content. The value of these studies and others is that by increasing hemoglobin levels, there is an enhancement of cellular metabolism and consequently, a positive change in the well-being of the person. The same holds true for the plants. There is a cellular enhancement and consequently an improvement in growth and productivity. By the time you talk lovingly to them too...look out!

If you're hungry for more technical data and studies done in the field of healing, I encourage you to read *Hands of Light* by Barbara Brennan and *Living the Therapeutic Touch* by Dolores Krieger.

In hands-on-healing (or "healing touch"), the assumption is made that as human beings we are made up of energy in a solid form, and surrounded by more of that same energy extending out around us in a more invisible form. This invisible energy surrounding us is called an energy field.

On a daily basis, we are continually engaged in an invisible energy exchange with our environment. You may recall places that made you feel wonderful just to be there, just as other places made you feel awful. Or, you've heard people say things like, "She gives me a lift," or "One minute with him and I feel absolutely drained." The responses vary from subtle to profound, to outrageous. Increasing your awareness of what's happening around you on an energy level means that you can deliberately enhance your own life and the lives of others.

Illness can be looked upon as having an energy imbalance, blockage, or deficit. We, as healers, can intentionally transfer energy to the ill person, promoting the restoration of harmony, balance and flow, as we enhance their well-being or "wholeness." Furthermore, the person who is ill can also "intentionally" draw healing energy into his/her own body, promoting health and revitalization.

The healing process itself can be likened to a dance—dancing until you become "one" with the dance or one with the healing energy. Or it can be described as a state of bliss that penetrates the very core of your being. When you are using the process to help someone, it's as if you begin to cycle a blissful state within yourself, and the healee has the option of "jumping in," catching the healing rhythm as you offer it. It reminds me of the way we used to jump rope with one another as kids. Our eyes would study the rope going 'round and 'round, our palms moving slightly as we sought a common rhythm. At the perfect moment, we'd "jump in." In healing, the process begins when the healee catches the rhythm and opts to "jump in."

The fascinating thing is that you don't even have to touch the person physically. This is especially valuable when working with burned patients. A repeated sweep of the hand through the person's energy field (unruffling) can mean the difference between pain and comfort. It even works right through casts, clothing and rubber gloves!

Just what are the effects of using this gentle technique? The energy exchange is known to:

- Accelerate healing, enhancing the body's natural ability to "self-correct."

- Reduce and often eliminate all pain.

- Relieve anxiety, replacing it with a sense of well-being and relaxation. (Some have coined this response a "drugless high!")

In the Orlando area, I've had a program underway in the Neonatal Intensive Care Unit of a local hospital. The nurses are using hands-on-healing techniques as a very normal extension of their nursing care. The results have been almost magical. As one nurse put it when treating premies (premature infants) hooked to monitoring equipment, "I could immediately see positive changes on the data coming from the machines, correlating to the same moment I began the treatment." It validated what she was also noting personally, that the "premie" was breathing much more easily and calming down. (How wonderful to have the *old* or ancient techniques validated by the *new* high-tech equipment!)

Other demonstrations of success include a spontaneous remission of a three-month case of thrush (fungal infection on the hard palate in the mouth) hours after a healing treatment. In a case of retrolentalfibroplasia (RLF), which is eye damage due to high levels of oxygen, the infant was taken down to surgery and surgery was canceled due to a "spontaneous remission of RLF." The nurse had given the infant a healing treatment the night before.

I have been delighted with the success I've seen in using healing touch on cardiac patients—even those who have backslid after bypass surgery and found that their arteries were clogged once again. As Naomi, a 74-year-old client put it, "I literally thought the jig was up. I would just have to live with daily pain and exhaustion, hoping nothing worse would happen." One treatment made an enormous improvement in her energy level. I taught her how to do a healing treatment on herself daily and techniques to use if pain occurs. Naomi also relaxes daily with a guided imagery meditation tape. In other words, she has learned that she is able to exert some control over her health and energy level. She has taken responsibility for her health. You may see her as you pass through the area...she's the one smiling as she takes her daily walks!

One more word about Naomi. While she was walking one day, she began to have angina (a painful spasm associated with the lack of oxygen to the heart muscle). She said, "Normally, I would have absolutely panicked. I was a few blocks from home and without medication. I merely slowed my pace and put my hand up to my heart, sending it healing energy. I arrived home in no time flat with nothing more than tired legs!"

I have used it successfully on countless back injuries, cancer patients, postoperative surgical patients, broken bones, carpal tunnel syndrome, eye injuries, sports injuries, angina, strokes, asthma, newborns (including premature infants), burns, and anxiety, just to name a few. My "patients" have included horses, dogs, cats, turtles, fish, plants...and anyone who will sit still long enough! "Life Force" has a marvelous way of enhancing all forms of life.

The bottom line in using healing touch is that it always works. I bet you're shocked! It just may not work in the way you thought it would. Whether you see a demonstration or not, there is always a positive benefit on some level...physical, emotional or spiritual. It may be that the energy merely offers an internal support to do needed work in one or more of those areas or it may be in laying the groundwork for future healing. This is something to explain to your ego when you are wandering away from a treatment feeling unsuccessful!

When we study the human body, we find all kinds of systems. There's a digestive system, nervous system, endocrine system, and more. Norman Cousins (author of *Anatomy of an Illness*) points out that not one medical text includes the one that might be placed right at the top of the list, "The Healing System"! Doesn't that have a nice ring to it? With our knowledge about healing today, this system would not only include the immune system but how body and mind interact to promote health. It would show the careful blend and orchestration of all the body's "systems" to maintain health. Literally billions of dollars are spent yearly on studying disease instead of studying health! How about visualizing future medical texts with two headings: "The Healing System," and, "What Causes Health?" It's a beginning!

Chapter 4

Reality...On An Energy Level!

Linda has a split personality. What's even more important is that one personality has diabetes. As Linda switches from one personality to the other, her pancreas alternates between functioning and non-functioning. The fascinating switch is apparently controlled by the personality...or by thought!

Equally fascinating are documented cases involving high blood pressure, severe allergies, epilepsy, rashes, warts, scars, color blindness, etc., appearing and disappearing as the personalities switch from one to the other.

On a cellular level, you are constantly responding to ongoing thoughts, including self-talk and visualizations or mental pictures. For example, imagine going to the kitchen and carefully cutting open a nice fresh lemon. Now, pick up a large piece of lemon and bite into it with all your might...that's it...slop around in all that juice and keep chewing! Did that get your salivary glands going? No lemon actually present, just the thought...bingo, lots of saliva!

Have you ever thought how fascinating "thoughts" are? They are actually energy held in space by the mind! This energy is peaking with creativity. The minute it even exists, it sets vibrations in motion with its very existence...dynamic and invisible, constantly shaping your existence and quality of life. Worth thinking about, wouldn't you say?

By now, we've all heard how healthy hugs are! But, have you noticed that some seem healthier than others? There's my favorite...the all out "bear hug." It's wide open, full of meaning, full of gusto! Then there's the "A-frame Hug," touching only at the shoulders or cheeks, elbows held close to the sides, and often accompanied by rapid light patting on your back!

There is an automatic exchange of energy in hugging that can enhance both persons. However, the magical ingredient that transforms an ordinary hug or an ordinary touch into something of much greater magnitude is intention! You guessed it—we're back to "thought"! Are you merely hugging, or are you sending that person some loving energy at the same time? The whole process lies in your thoughts.

In doing healing, there are several ways in which intention enhances the process:

- The first is your basic *intention to help or heal.* This is the bottom line in any healing.

- The second is your *intention that your work be for the highest good of all concerned.* This refers to both you and the healee, and the fact that you want each of you to come away all the better for having had the experience.

- Third, energy actually flows with intention. To put it quite simply, you *intend that the energy flow...* and it does! Just like that!

- Fourth, with regard to the specific areas of the body that you decide to work on, you *intend that the energy be unlimited.* That is, that it go wherever it needs to go, and in precisely the right amount to re-establish harmony and balance in the body. While your attention may be drawn to a certain area or specific symptoms, the real problem could very well be elsewhere. You might think of the energy as politely awaiting direction from you to proceed. With this type of greater awareness in your intention, it's not uncommon to treat one ailment and have others also disappear! Now, doesn't that last version sound like more fun? I thought so! I "intended" it that way!

I used to worry about whether I was supposed to move my hand clockwise or counter-clockwise when doing certain techniques. Oooooh, what if I were to do it wrong? I learned many "always'" and "nevers" as they related to healing. On more than one occasion I met up with others who were quite successful doing it exactly the opposite way. What we each had in common was our "intention."

The healing process is a continually creative one. There are no perfect techniques to "always" use. If during one of your treatments you couldn't remember a technique to use, but had the intention to help or heal for the highest good, you'd be all set. To merely allow life force to flow with the proper intention is really what this is all about. Couple that with your intuitiveness, and you're all set to invent and create as you flow with life force. *Intention actually over-rides technique. Energy follows your intention!*

Chapter 5

Getting Started

It's time to suit up! It's very important to dress for the occasion. The outfit that is most appropriate and fashionable for healing is a beautiful shimmering white light. One that not only surrounds you and extends out past your body, but which fills every inch of you inside as well.

It's very easy to do this with *breath*. Draw in shimmering white (divine) light as you inhale...*hold your breath momentarily* at the top of your inhalation, filling every inch inside you with white light. As you exhale through your mouth, *expand* the light outwards, sending it right through your skin and creating a cocoon-like buffer all around you. You fill up...then expand! An additional reason that I enjoy this version is for the cleansing it facilitates as it expands. I can feel it pushing out negative energy as well.

Yet another way is merely to visualize white light in and around you. If you are not a visual person and can't imagine a white light, then just declare that it is now filling and surrounding you. (That "covers you," so to speak!)

You also help the healee to suit up properly for the occasion. Merely visualize (or declare) that he is filled and surrounded with white light as well.

The white light is unique in that it is *semi-permeable*... letting in only love and positive energy, but all negativity is unable to penetrate. It's an outfit in which you can easily work through, sensing what you need to sense for your work, but protecting yourself and the healee from unwanted negative energy. Once you fill and surround yourself in white light, you do not need to continue concentrating on it to keep it there. It remains in place quite nicely!

Without the white light or a similar precaution, you are leaving yourself wide open for "picking up" negative clutter. You can even pick up a symptom, although not the disease or problem itself. For example, without shielding yourself in any way, you send healing energy to someone with a sore knee and *come away with a sore knee yourself!* The white light could have prevented this from transferring. In other words, you wouldn't have ended up wearing the same problem yourself.

I have a friend whose little dog Max had been hit by a car. His right hip was injured. She immediately began working on Max who responded very well to the healing. My friend's delight didn't last long, however. She quickly realized that now her right hip was in terrible pain! Since then, she has always used the white light and "the case of the traveling symptom" has never re-occurred!

There are many ways to incorporate the white light into your daily life. Shopping malls are filled to the brim with negativity. You may notice that after only a few minutes' exposure to the environment there, your energy level takes a rapid dive. Using the white light before you arrive can prevent the problem. You may want to use it before going to work or before the kids come home!

I also enjoy sending white light to others...giving them some help in dealing with life. For example, I bestow it along with a blessing to hitchhikers, stray dogs and cats, people I see anywhere who seem to be struggling with life, and even my son or husband as they leave for the day. Or I surround the car or plane that loved ones are traveling in. It's a very useful and down-to-earth technique. Besides, you look great in white light...definitely a fashion statement.

The Connection...A Balancing Act

Let's see now...you have your "outfit," and your intention, and now you're grounded! Webster's Dictionary describes this as "preventing the pilot from flying!" The purpose of grounding is to keep you connected to the earth's energy as you experience universal energy, so you don't "space out" during the work. (If you leave, who's going to take care of the healee?)

The idea is to feel a sense of balance. You're in a delightful spot, holding the centermost point in sensing your connection with the earth, and simultaneously sensing your connection with the universe. No fair playing favorites and taking in more of one without an equal awareness of the other!

You can practice this state using a short guided imagery. Sit comfortably, feet flat on the floor. Take a long deep breath in through your nose and let it all out through your mouth. Bring your awareness to your lower back, legs and feet. Imagine long extensions projecting from your feet and penetrating deep within the earth, like the roots of an oak tree. Enjoy that feeling for a moment. Now, imagine the energy of the earth, flowing up through your body and out through the top of your head, into the universe. After experiencing that for a few moments, allow the light energy from the universe to enter through the crown of your head, harmoniously blending earth energy with universal energy right inside your body. What a nice blend!

Remaining On Center While Healing

Ahhh, you say, on the center of what? Along with centering *above* with *below,* it's important to find a spot mentally that is quite "present." By that I mean that you are not leaning mentally backwards into the past or forward into the future, but you are totally centered here and now. This means consciously drawing your awareness into the core of your "being"...and I might add, then operating from an "intuitive witness state." It is a state in which you become totally present with the healee and establish a very definite soul-to-soul connection. In the beginning, it is quite helpful to remain quiet while you work in order to experience this state of consciousness. I have found that I can easily remain on center even while chatting with the client. Part of me stays right on center...kind of on "automatic pilot," while the other part chats. I've learned to do it that way out of necessity, since some clients prefer to talk during their treatments. It's great training for learning to go about your daily life...on center!

There are many meditative processes that can assist you in practicing the centered state. I suggest, for a starter, that you just sit quietly with your eyes closed, and focus on your breathing. Become your breath. Be the air moving in and out. This is practice being totally present with you. If your mind wanders, just lovingly note, "Ahh, my mind wandered," and bring yourself back to center. No fury about it. Just note it and begin again. You may even want some soft meditative music in the background. Practicing the centered state allows you to quickly clear your mind of chatter and become totally focused on the healing at hand. It helps you to become a clearer channel for the healing energy.

In the next chapter you will see that you've just learned the first step in healing: *Centering, Shielding, and Intending.*

Chapter 6

Six Steps In Healing

The Triple Awareness Breath (Step One)

You now have the start-up procedure for healing:

- Centering (including grounding)
- Shielding (white light)
- Intending (setting the intention that only the highest good be done)

With practice the above awarenesses become as easy and as automatic as putting your shoes on. Although each one was described in length, you can easily learn to assimilate all three into the time it takes for one breath. I call it the "triple awareness breath." It is a meditative spot that becomes your "mind-set" for healing. Try it with me slowly. Center and pull in the white light as you inhale, expand the white light and intend that "only the highest good be done" as you exhale. You're getting it!

The Scan (Step Two...Optional)

Let's see now... you've just taken your "triple awareness breath" and I suppose you think you are ready to "roll with the flow," so to speak. Not so fast!... First, I want to introduce you to an option called "scanning."

As I explained earlier, you have an *energy field* that extends out several inches from your body. Scanning is done by gently moving your hands through that field as you watch for any perceived "differences." It's like *listening with your hands.* Often perceptions of heat, cold, static electricity, congestion, pulsations, etc. can be felt. These cues are merely areas that call to your attention.

In the first chapter, you may remember that this was the very exercise in which I felt nothing! I continued to practice scanning thinking that eventually the sensitivity would develop. Desperation grew and I became obsessed about increasing the sensitivity in my hands and becoming a "feeling healer"! I tried everything from declaring, allowing, bargaining, meditating, praying, to throwing my hands up in despair and releasing. Still nothing. However, at the same time I was seeing more and more success with every treatment.

I have since learned that we all have four psychic "gifts" that we use for experiencing life. These are *feeling, seeing, hearing,* and *knowing.* They are referred to as our "gift order" due to the fact that each of us has our own unique sequence. Your first "gift" would be the style with which you most easily sense and assimilate life. Obviously, *feeling* is not my number one gift!

You can even listen for the person's orientation in their speech. A visual person would tend to say, "I see what you mean." An auditory person would say, "I hear ya! I hear ya!" A knowing person would say, "I know what you mean." While a feeling person would say, "I feel exactly the same way."

The important thing is that you allow yourself to unfold in your own style. One is not better than another. The field of hands-on-healing seems to attract those who are intuitively sensitive with their hands, so the odds are that you will find your hands are able to sense all kinds of differences when scanning. If not...lighten up! It is not the sole criterion for being successful in this work. You'll find it just as easy to incorporate any of the other three psychic gifts into your personal style of healing.

I include the technique of scanning as an optional technique to develop. It's like having another radio station to play. With practice, those with sensitive hands can detect energy imbalances and problem areas. They can tell when balance and flow have returned just by feeling.

You've probably guessed by now that I personally omit the scanning step! But, don't be hasty in deciding whether you are a "feeler" or a "non-feeler." Gently allow yourself to unfold as you stay open to all possibilities. Continue to practice sensing with your hands but keep in mind the cues might be coming through other avenues as well. It's a wonderful *new you* that you are getting to know!

Are you ready? It's time to practice!

Before scanning, it's good to prepare your hands so that they are more sensitive. (Hopefully, you've actually washed your hands before the treatment!) Stretch or spread your fingers as widely apart from each other as possible. Hold that stretch for about fifteen seconds and then relax.

The scan itself takes only about thirty to sixty seconds from beginning to end, head to foot. Work with relaxed hands and remember to keep breathing as you work. We tend to hold our breath when concentrating on something new. Scan approximately 3-5 inches from the body. Remember that there are no right or wrong perceptions. You are merely scanning for *differences or areas that call to your attention.* No need to scan a particular area repeatedly in order to validate what you feel. Learn to go with your first impression...each time you pass your hand through the field, you've changed it. You've heard how important first impressions are!

Note: If you don't have a partner to practice on, scan your own body. Scan pets. Scan plants. Scan any live thing...but scan!

Since any other contact with the healee's energy field changes the field itself, *scanning must be the first thing you do.* Then continue on with whatever you'd like.

During this or any other phase of the healing, be aware of "intuitive messages" that might be floating into your awareness. Keep in mind that even though it sounds like your same old "internal voice" speaking, you may often be receiving thoughts that are of a higher level...some call it "guidance." So get busy *suspecting* that maybe, just maybe, this might be important!

Unruffling...The Fun Step! (Step Three)

While unruffling is a valid intervention technique (see Step Four, page 43). It deserves to be included as a consistent step in every healing treatment, prior to all other techniques.

Unruffling is done with a sweeping movement of the hands, a few inches away from the body, usually from head to foot. It involves faster, longer sweeps than in the scanning process. There is no attempt to "sense" anything with the hands. You are merely clearing "clutter" out of the energy field. Cleaning house, so to speak.

Several things can be accomplished with unruffling:

- It accelerates the effectiveness of all other work by clearing the way to "let healing in."

- It helps to redistribute areas of energy "overload" with the areas where it is lacking.

- It clears congestion in the energy field promoting a sense of calm or well-being.

- In areas of energy stagnation, it frees up the healee's energy so that flow is restored and balance can return.

Irritable? Having a generally harried day? Is that what's bothering you? Well, for heaven's sake, unruffle yourself! The picture of that alone should bring a chuckle or two! The process of that alone will create an instant change in how you feel. Presto, you feel lighter. Life seems easier.

One of the reasons it feels good to unruffle is thought to have to do with ionization. Ions are atoms having a negative or positive electrical charge from gaining or losing an electron. While positive ions are associated with headaches and irritability, an abundance of negative ions brings about feelings of well-being and comfort. This is one time when it's good to have an abundance of the negative! With the sweep of the hand, positive ions are moved out of the energy field and replaced by negative ions.

Perhaps you've heard of "negative ionizers" which are devices used in restaurants, doctors' offices and other public places to give you a settled, comfortable feeling. They often look like inconspicuous little black boxes. Other versions are seen hanging from the ceiling looking like microphones. The benefit is that they increase the negative ion content in the air, which in turn, promotes an "anti-frantic" or calm atmosphere. Negative ions have also been shown to promote accelerated healing in patients with severe burns.

The ocean, waterfalls, and mountains are areas in nature where negative ions seem to be naturally abundant. It feels great just to hang out there. You can capture some of that feeling for yourself just with the sweep of your hand! Brush those positive ions away and make room for all the wonderful negative ions. See why I call this the "Fun Step"?

Intervention Techniques
...or what you do with what you've found!
(Step Four)

Sooo, you scanned the healee and found areas that called to your attention, did you? Whether you picked up cues on the scan or not, it's now time to roll with the flow! The idea is to promote balance and harmony in the healee. But how do we know what to do?

I must have you picture me at this same point in my own journey as a healer. We were taught to modulate or to adjust the healee's energy patterns by responding to the cues picked up in the scan. We were to bring it back into balance by treating it with the opposing pattern. In other words, if we felt heat on one side of the body and coolness on the other, we intentionally sent its opposite until an evenness in temperature was felt on both sides. But remember, *I wasn't feeling a thing!* This was an extremely frustrating exercise for me personally.

My version became quite a simple one out of necessity. I humorously describe the process as one composed of "stop, go, and bless!" We were cautioned not to overload the healee with energy and shown how to sense the moment when a blocked energy center (chakra) actually reopened. None of this was a reality for me. I watched as others delighted in their new-found sensitivity.

What appeared as a handicap in the beginning, turned into a treasured gift and one of the greatest a-ha's I've ever experienced. While still eagerly anticipating the day in which I would join ranks of many of my students and peers who could sense so keenly with their hands, I was struck one afternoon with the reality of the situation. I had been so busy waiting to become a "feeling healer" that I had nearly missed a truth staring me right in the face...the reason my own version was quite successful.

Out of necessity, I had leaned on the divine aspect of the energy to fill in where I could not...Lord knows I didn't know what the healee needed where! There was the A-ha! *The divine energy has a "knowingness" all its own and can be intentionally released to do the highest good in the process!* And all along, I thought perhaps it was just having mercy on me until I caught up with the others!

The trick seems to be in getting out of the way and allowing the process to be all it can be. (Unlimited!) If we don't place a limited focus on our work, could it develop in a bigger way, beyond what is apparent in our consciousness at this point? For example, when I'm working say, on a sore wrist, I intentionally ask that the energy go wherever else it is needed as well, including all levels of awareness...physical, emotional, and spiritual.

But my version is only one style. Perhaps you are keenly sensitive with your hands and raring to go when it comes to handling what you've found in the scan. The basic goal is to re-establish flow where there are blockages and to restore harmony and balance to the body. I've already mentioned treating the cues with their opposites. If you find an area that seems to be pulsating, you intentionally send energy to quiet it. *Remember, energy follows your "intention."* If you find an area of congestion, you attempt to sweep it away or disperse it. If you perceive an energy deficit, you intentionally refuel it. A good rule of thumb is to stay with the area until the cues cease or you sense that balance has returned.

But, it isn't enough to mechanically even-out the cues with their opposites; equally as important is an increased awareness of intuitiveness or higher guidance that is at your service. You don't think you have intuition? Sure you do! For some it comes as clearly heard messages; for others it comes as visual pictures or just a subtle urge to follow through in a certain way. But it is there so watch for it and use it! Start suspecting that maybe, just maybe, this isn't just more of your ordinary thoughts or mental images. Allow that part of you to unfold. You'll have a new friend and support system to enjoy in all of your life, not just in healing.

Ahhh yes... on to the flow itself! A very simple but profound process! The key here again is intention. You merely *intend* that the energy flow... and bingo, it does! I bet you thought it would be much more difficult than that, huh! There is no need for anything dramatic or flashy, no need to work yourself into a lather. A very easy way to experience the flow is to practice drawing the energy in through the crown of your head from your personal *Source* as you inhale... and sending it out through the palms of your hands as you exhale. It cycles with each breath but works much like a siphon. Once you get it started, it flows effortlessly and fluidly needing no concentration on your part.

In my mind's eye, I personally see this same process as energy coming in through my crown in the form of *light*. As I exhale, it flows out through the palms of my hands, lighting up the corresponding area on the healee. It's like having a flashlight beaming from each palm, and in essence *touching with light*. I visualize the process as lighting up dark and stagnant areas, and in turn re-establishing flow and balance.

Take a moment to experience this flow for yourself. First of all, take your *triple awareness breath* in which you center, shield, and intend. Unruffle your chest and abdomen and place one hand on your heart, the other on your solar plexus (the area just under your rib cage). Now inhale deeply through your nose as you intentionally pull energy in through your crown... pull, pull, pull it in as you inhale (good)... and release the energy through the palms of your hands as you exhale through your mouth. Continue cycling the energy with your breath. Just like a siphon, once the flow is well established it self-propels on its own. You ultimately enjoy an effortless flow of healing energy. Give it permission to go wherever it needs to go and to be all it can be for your highest good! By the way, whether you feel anything or not, know that it's flowing and that wonderful things are happening! As with anything, the more you practice the better you get at it and the easier it becomes. This exercise is a marvelous way to say "thank you" to you, to celebrate all that you are!

There will be more specific intervention techniques to follow. But for now, realize that if you did nothing more than intentionally flow with the healing energy, you would have tapped into the profound!

Grounding The Healee (Step Five)

Note: For simplification, the healee will be referred to as "he" in the generic sense.

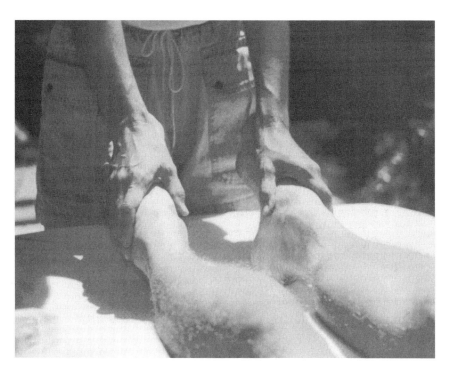

Figure 6.1: Grounding

I've mentioned the importance of *grounding yourself* when you work. However, step five refers to *grounding the healee* after a treatment of any length; sessions in which the healee slides into a very deep state of relaxation. This level of relaxation can give the sensation of "floating" afterwards (unsafe for driving, etc.).

You can ground the healee merely by holding his feet or shoulders for a moment (see Figure 6.1). It also helps to have him drink water. Besides its grounding ability, good water intake after a treatment helps to flush out toxins that are released in the healing process. The healee might as well get started on the water consumption and ground at the same time!

Terminating The Treatment (Step Six)

When do you quit? You stop when everything is quiet on the home front. The busy-ness or activity that you were feeling has quieted. A sense of balance seems to be restored. Or, when merely energizing a person whose energy is depleted, perhaps you no longer feel the *drawing* sensation in your hands, a sensation that feels as if the healee is pulling in the energy. Also, listen for inner guidance as to when it's time to quit.

I have found that it's important to have a clear-cut method of breaking the connection between you (the healer) and the healee. Otherwise, there is a certain amount of "connectedness" that can continue for some time which acts as a drain on your own energy. It will gradually fade away on its own, but it pays to be definite about it. You can either just mentally declare that you are now through and "disconnect," or take the side of your hand, palm toward you, and "slice" down the front of your torso, breaking all connection (see Figure 6.2). I find the latter simple and very effective. I do it immediately after the treatment just before washing my hands.

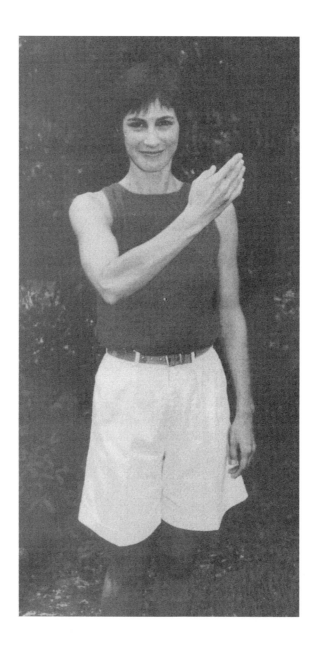

Figure 6.2: Disconnecting

In summary, there are six steps in healing:

1. Triple Awareness Breath

2. Scanning (Optional)

3. Unruffling

4. Intervention Techniques (Intuitive Work)

5. Grounding The Healee

6. Terminating The Treatment

Chapter 7

Specific Intervention Techniques

This is where you allow your intuitive skills to blossom and intend that the energy be all that it can be. It is a totally creative process and hopefully one that aims at simplicity at the same time.

The following is a group of techniques that are ideal for use during a full healing treatment. Or, you can use any of them by themselves for localized or brief treatments...but be sure you still include your *intention* and the *triple awareness breath* before beginning.

The Energy Flow

I've already discussed the benefit of the flow of energy itself. If you did nothing more than place your hands on the healee and intentionally let the energy flow, you would have offered a profound gift!

Unruffling

Along with using unruffling to soothe and calm or to clear the way to receive the energy, it does wonders for a number of specific problems. This is the technique of choice for soothing and healing burns. It has brought tremendous relief to severely burned patients who were previously unrelieved by pain medications. Unruffling also works wonders for any areas of congestion, whether all the congestion is solely in the energy field or physically manifested as in the case of lung congestion. Happy sweeping!

Massage

Along with unruffling, massage is yet another way to encourage the body to let the healing energy in. In areas where the energy is blocked, massage seems to help restore the flow once again.

This doesn't have to be fancy...the key here once again is the "intent." Are you absentmindedly massaging...or are you *massaging!* You'll often get an ahhh with the second kind. I find that doing it *slowly, lovingly, and with purpose* seems to accomplish more. You want to work WITH the tissue, not try to force it. You can either massage right through clothing or if the situation permits, you can get the old almond oil out and do an oil massage. You can even energize the oil for healing, adding even another dimension to your work! Merely hold the bottle of oil between your hands and let the energy flow into the oil. This only takes a few minutes.

Naturally, if the area in need of healing is infected, contused, or freshly injured, massage would not be appropriate or indicated. This is the beauty of hands-on-healing. It can be done without touching the skin at all, making it the ideal treatment of choice for all conditions where massage is not feasible.

Massage therapists have a perfect opportunity to blend healing right in with their entire massage. I have found that as long as I keep some movement going while directing energy, even a very slow rocking movement with my hands, no one grows concerned that the massage has stopped; no one questions the treatment being given. (I'm talking very s-l-o-w—like the rhythm of ocean tide flowing in and out.) The blending of healing energy with massage offers the ultimate in body/mind and spirit enhancement! The client can easily feel the difference, and the therapist comes away energized instead of fatigued. Talk about a win-win experience!

Sooo, consider paving the way for other healing techniques with massage!

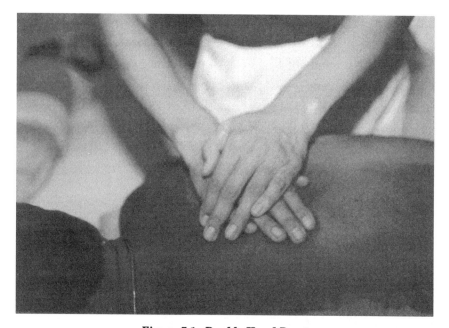

Figure 7.1: Double Hand Boost

Double Hand Boost

Nurses, massage therapists and just plain *people helping people* seem to have one thing in common: there never is enough time! The double hand boost emerged in my quest for ways to get better results in less time. The pain was relieved faster if I placed one hand on top of the other over the problem area, rather than two hands side by side (Figure 7.1). My experience seems to support the expression that two hands are better than one! Try it out for yourself when working on localized painful areas.

Laser

Not only can we intentionally direct energy from the palms of our hands, but from the very tips of our fingers as well. Energy just naturally extends from your fingertips. Now imagine what you can do with that! For example, you can point your fingers straight into a painful area, and with your fingers lightly touching the surface of the skin, "laser" the area (Figure 7.2). I often rock my hands (slowly) back and forth, changing the angle in which the energy is entering the body. This works great for sore spots and sore joints.

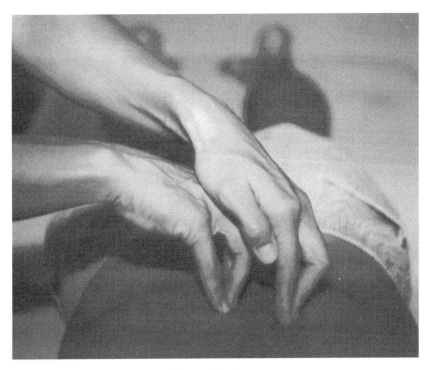

Figure 7.2: Laser

Ultrasound

This name was coined by Janet Mentgen, a wonderful teacher and friend of mine, in Colorado. It has been one of the most effective techniques I know for relieving pain and for getting things moving. I tried it out on a friend of mine with a sore muscle the day after I learned it. Four minutes later, there was no pain! That got my attention, and this technique has been a favorite ever since.

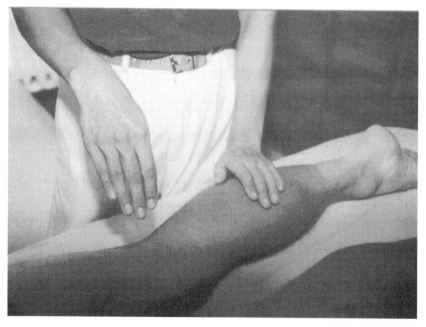

Figure 7.3: Ultrasound

Ultrasound uses the same principle as lasering. You use the energy that naturally extends from your fingertips as tools. One hand is placed on the healee, adjacent to the painful area. Now, point the fingers of your opposite hand straight into the focal area and move your hand in a circular motion just above the skin (Figure 7.3). It's the movement that seems to be important. I generally make clockwise circles but I've seen wonderful results from those using counterclockwise circles or even a side-to-side motion. I have found this to be even more effective when using the double hand boost beforehand.

The Siphon

A commonly held thought in working with energy is that we think of the left hand "receiving" and the right hand "giving." The siphon is based on this philosophy. First, the left hand is used to siphon (receive) toxins, pain or whatever needs to leave the body. Then the right hand is used to replenish the same area with healing energy (or give healing energy). In reality, you can *intentionally* use either hand to give or receive, so don't get excited!

You begin by placing your left hand on the problem area. Your right hand is positioned down at your side and slightly away from your body (Figure 7.4). Intentionally begin receiving or "siphoning" the pain, toxins, etc., from the area with your left hand and have it exit through your right hand. Your right hand is "giving" it away. I intentionally add that the negative contents siphoned off turns into positive energy for the universe as it exits!

You may feel a lot of action in one or both hands after you hold this position awhile. Wait until it quiets down. This could take some time. When all sensations have ceased, replace your left hand with your right. This time the *right* hand is on the problem area and your *left* hand is held up in the air, similar to when you raised your hand to ask a question in school (Figure 7.5). Your left hand is now receiving healing energy and your right hand is giving it to the healee...filling the void with healing energy.

Specific Intervention Techniques 59

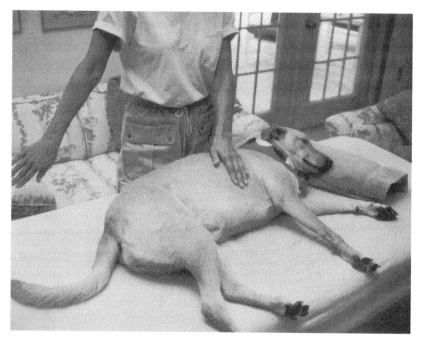

Figure 7.4: First Position (Siphon)

I found that I was uncomfortable with the thought of all that "stuff" flowing through me as the healer, and developed an additional version that I find more desirable. I create an imaginary tube through which the unwanted material can flow so that I don't have to experience it as it travels through me. Naturally, I don't mind experiencing the healing energy during the second step!

This technique takes more time than some of the others but it's very effective. It seems to be quite effective in removing deep-seated pain.

Remember, *the left hand receives*. First it receives the unwanted "stuff," then it receives the healing energy. *The right hand gives*. First it gives away what you've siphoned, then it gives the healing energy to the healee! And since *your intention overrides your technique*, you could even reverse the hand positions and still be successful. Isn't this easy?

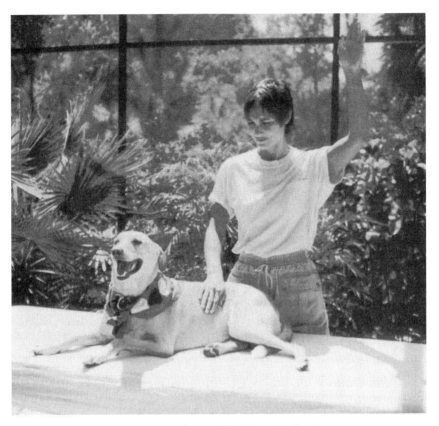

Figure 7.5: Second Position (Siphon)

Fluffing The Aura

Fluffing the aura (energy field around the body) seems to lift one's spirits. It seems to work well on anyone with depression. (Perhaps because like unruffling, it offers light-hearted entertainment for the beholder.) It is also done with the sweep of the hands, but all motion is in an upward sweep. For clients having a "down" day, I normally include unruffling first, then end the treatment by fluffing the aura.

Reflexology...
The Painless Way!

Remember when I said to listen to your inner guidance and more inspiration will come to you? Well, this is a creation that came to me when I was doing foot reflexology.

Reflexology deals with the principle that there are reflex points on your hands and feet which directly correspond to glands, organs, and parts of the body. You can enhance the wellness of all of these body parts by working the precise spot on the foot or hand with your thumb or finger. This can often be *painful*. The reflex points have been referred to as the "Oh, yes!" points because when asked if the area is tender, the client literally belts out, "Oh, yes!" I loved the theory and the results it seemed to produce, but hated causing pain in the process.

One day I was working on a good friend who had been diagnosed as having an ovarian cyst. The cyst was tender to palpate and the corresponding ovarian point on her ankle was also extremely tender. The idea came to me to send energy at the reflex point on the foot rather than to put painful pressure on it. I first used a double hand boost over the point and followed with ultrasound on the same area. Within minutes the tenderness in her reflex point disappeared. Upon palpating the right ovary again, no pain! A CAT scan a few days later revealed that the cyst had decreased by 50 per cent!

Since then, I have utilized the reflex points on the foot to relieve or heal problems elsewhere in the body, but I do it *painlessly with energy* instead of finger pressure. Intention, the mother of invention!

The Back Package
(Including The Hopi Indian Technique)

The "back package" is made up of the following:

- Massage
- The Thumb Walk
- The Hopi Indian Technique
- Ultrasound

I have found this to be an extremely effective combination for painful backs. Profound changes have occurred even when students were practicing the techniques for the very first time. One workshop participant excitedly related that he could now comfortably bend over and place his hands flat on the floor. For two years prior to that his wife had helped him with his shoes each morning because he couldn't begin to reach his own feet!

Massage

The value of massage as a means of paving the way for other techniques has already been discussed. I just want to add that it seems to be of particular benefit in this package because it encourages the back muscles to relax and stimulates the flow of energy. Again, you may do this right through clothing or grab the old almond oil and go for it! In most cases, especially when there is pain present, *slow deliberate massage* seems to develop a sense of trust and bring about faster relaxation.

The Thumb Walk

This technique is one I like to include for treating any back problem, being sensitive to the amount of pressure being exerted at the site of any injury. It does wonders for the back itself, is very relaxing, and it also energizes each of the spinal nerves that connect with various body organs, enhancing the well-being of each. It's like a "mini tune-up" for your body!

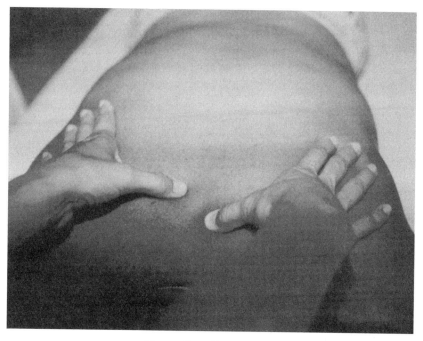

Figure 7.6: Thumb Walk

To begin, stand at the head of the table with the healee *lying face down* (Figure 7.6). (If no face cradle is available, a rolled towel can be placed under the healee's forehead, along with a pillow under the chest area. This not only allows a comfortable space for the face to rest but also promotes proper alignment. Elevating the feet with a pillow underneath relaxes the low back and also offers more comfort in this position.) Place one open hand on each side of the upper spine, palms down, thumbs toward the spinal column. Feel for a nice little groove between each pair of adjacent vertebrae. You'll find your thumb fits nicely in the groove. As you place one thumb in the first groove, slowly rotate the tip of your thumb in a tiny circular motion (either direction) as you press firmly. While that thumb is working, your other thumb hunts for the corresponding groove on the opposite side of the spine. Once you have found it, switch the rotation to that thumb. Then repeat the process, alternating as you do the *thumb walk* down the spine. Happy trails!

The Hopi Indian Technique

Ahh, the Hopi Indian! This is my all time favorite back technique. It is believed to have originated from a Hopi medicine man who shared it with the Reverend Rudy Noel of Denver. I received it indirectly and by the time I saw it in its original version, I realized that my technique was slightly different. For a while, I contemplated changing. However, eventually I realized that it was extremely effective just as I was doing it. Here's where *intention* comes up again! I intended this technique to free up the blocks in the back as I worked, therefore, it usually did. At any rate, here is my version.

With the healee still prone (face down), stand to one side. I generally begin on the healee's left side.

Here are four positions:

- First Position: Begin at the base of the neck, near or on the first thoracic vertebrae. The first position is nothing more than a double hand boost on that spot (Figure 7.7). This is light work...don't lean! Hold the position for a few minutes, or until all cues you might be experiencing cease.

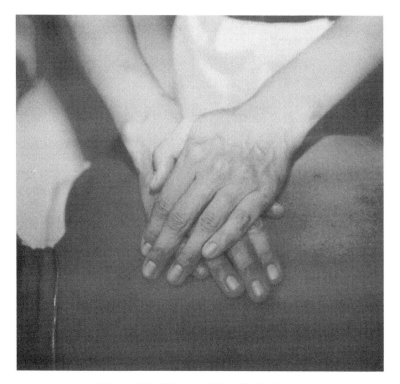

Figure 7.7: First and Fourth Positions

- Second Position: Without breaking contact, *slowly slide your hands* into the "laser" position on the same area. Place the fingertips of one hand on the far side of the spine, fingertips of the other hand are on the closer or proximal side of the spine. Your fingers are relaxed. All four fingers on each hand (without the thumbs) line up in a row on each side, parallel to the spine. They are *lightly* touching the skin. Your *wrists are touching each other,* making a little "A-frame" figure over the spine (Figure 7.8). Just hold this position, essentially using the "laser" technique, and intending that the energy flow through your fingers.

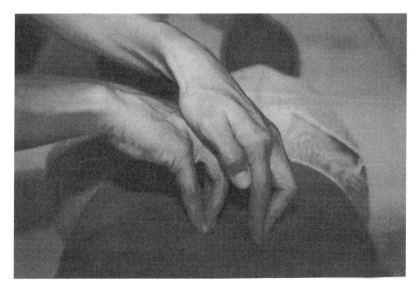

Figure 7.8: Second Position

Many times at this point, I begin to sense "needles and pins" sensations in my fingers. It's not uncommon for the healee to feel sensations as well. Some even feel unusual sensations in their feet and swear that you must be using something other than just your fingertips! Move on to the next position when all sensations or "cues" cease, or, if you aren't sensing a thing, move on as you intuitively feel ready. Know that it is working even if you feel nothing!

- <u>Third Position</u>: Slowly slide into the third position. This is the one that may feel the most awkward, but you will easily adapt to it. (I know how flexible and flowing you are in life!) Place the thumbs of both hands on the proximal side of the spine (the side closest to you). Directly across from each thumb, but on the opposite side of the spine, place each middle finger. As you do this, use what's called the *flats* of your fingers...bend the last section of both fingers and thumbs so that they lie mostly horizontal to the healee's back (see Figures 7.9 and 7.10).

Specific Intervention Techniques 67

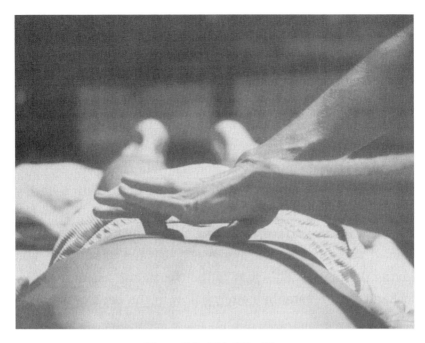

Figure 7.9: Third Position

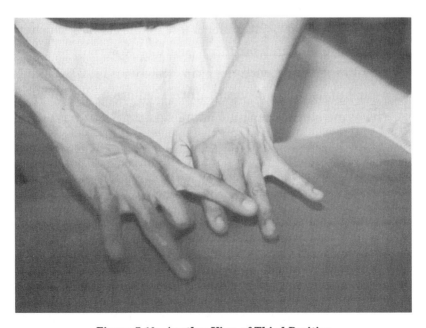

Figure 7.10: Another View of Third Position

While holding the third position (the one that's getting easier by the minute!), mentally imagine that your fingers have "extensions" going under the spine, connecting each finger with the thumb on the same hand. Press in slightly as you hold this position, and wait for a feeling of connection between the fingers and thumbs...as if a slight current is running from one to the other. If you don't sense the connection, just wait a bit and then continue right on with the process. Whether you sense the connection or not, continue on by pushing down with additional pressure into the tissue, and immediately pull your fingers up and off the skin surface, breaking the contact. (This resembles some of the quick upward moves Liberace used to do while playing the piano!) This part of the treatment seems to pull out blockages and reestablish energy flow in the back.

- <u>Fourth Position</u>: Immediately after breaking contact in the third position, return your hands to the same area...sealing the process with a double hand boost. Remain in that position for a few moments. Notice that you begin and end with this position. Now, without breaking contact with the skin, slowly and lovingly slide your hands to the adjacent untreated area...and repeat the same steps. Continue doing this until you have treated the entire spine.

I literally did this for 1-2 years without sensing a thing in the entire process, yet I had tremendous results with bad backs!

Recently, a friend told me that she had been quite successful using the Hopi Indian Technique on other areas of the body. She had even used it on the arch of the foot, which in Reflexology corresponds to the back. She found that utilizing the Hopi Indian Technique on these reflex points was also effective in relieving back problems. See? As you flow with life force, keep listening, keep creating! In an area as small as the arch, an area that corresponds to the entire spine, a lot of ground is covered just by doing "one little Indian!"

Ultrasound

The last step in the back package is ultrasound. Place one hand on the healee, and move the other in circles above the skin as you do the ultrasound up and down the spine. This seems to add just the right finishing touch!

The back package can facilitate a lot of change. As with all treatments, be sure to remind the healee to *drink plenty of water.* Many toxins are released in the process and need to be flushed out of the body.

It's important to realize that you may not see a change in the healee's symptoms until later that day or even the next day. I instruct clients that this work continues even after they leave, and to continue to watch for positive changes. Many of the changes will amaze both of you! It is extremely common to have the problem totally cleared in just a few hours. Your role, if you care to accept it, is to get your ego out of the way and detach yourself from the outcome!

Boosting And Balancing The Chakras

(This is a simple procedure but takes some explaining!)

Ever heard of "chakras"? (Pronounced like "shock-rahs"...among the humorous mispronunciations are Sheekras, Chokers, and Shockers!) In Sanskrit the word chakra means "wheel of light." Some describe each as a spinning wheel of energy located at strategic points along the ventral (front) part of the spine as well as the forehead and crown. Each radiates light energy *forward and upwards* to the next chakra.

Other versions have described the chakras as flowers. When the chakra is open and flowing, all the petals are open with energy emanating. I like the petal version!

When you hear someone discussing chakras, sometimes called energy centers, they are generally referring to the seven major chakras, although there are about 122 minor ones as well. The minor chakras we will be using are located at the major joints in the arms and legs (see Figure 7.11).

You will find different versions of chakras in different books. Some clairvoyants have described distinct colors for each of the seven major chakras. You will also find varying information as to what color each one tends to be. Some authorities list only six major chakras while others list seven or eight. Pick a version…any version! (It's your reality so pick the one you enjoy!) You'll have a tool that's invaluable.

Many people get quite excited about chakras and have many "always'" and "nevers" in discussing them. For centuries they have been a major focus for the seekers of higher spiritual growth. Again, they are tools and you can use them to achieve a variety of results. In this case, I will focus on the part they can play in facilitating healing and "wholeness."

What's the importance of these little flowers? They are a focus for restoring balance to your body. By knowing the location of each one you can deliberately use them to enhance the healing process. Some healers can actually sense individual chakras as they scan with their hands. (If you're unable to feel them…you're just fine. Hang in there!)

As well as affecting the well-being of the body as a whole, each chakra also has its own individual "mission" or reason for existence. For example, the fifth chakra, located in the throat, is there to assist with expression…the sixth chakra, located in the

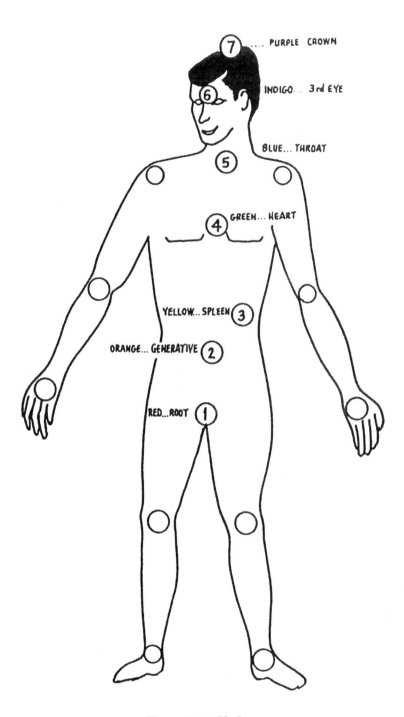

Figure 7.11: Chakras

forehead (also called the third eye), has to do with insight and inspiration. To energize or help open a chakra means that you are also promoting growth in its specific field of expertise! Each chakra is also directly related to an endocrine gland or organ, and when you enhance the chakra, the corresponding organ or gland is also enhanced. An excellent reference for more information regarding chakras is *Wheels of Light* by Rosalyn L. Bruyere.

A healthy open chakra dances full circle in a clockwise spin...clockwise as if it is the face of the clock. When all chakras are what we call "open" and balanced, there is a state of well-being and harmony. The area surrounding the chakras (including internal organs) derives health benefits from the openness as well. Likewise, when a chakra is blocked, the surrounding area is being compromised due to lack of energy flow.

There are varying degrees of "open-ness" in the petals. You might think of a blocked chakra as a tight flower bud that unfolds into full bloom as you enhance the chakra with energy. Chakras are frequently blocking and unfolding as you go about your day experiencing things emotionally. Surgery or trauma can cause the associated chakras to block. In a state of health, chakras self-correct on their own.

As you become more aware of body energies, you will become more attuned to when you are "open and flowing" and when you are blocked in certain areas. Consequently, you can personally feel the difference (and do something about it) when you have a case of the "tight petals!" A good example of a blocked chakra nearly everyone has experienced is the nausea, or butterflies, before speaking in front of an audience.

You will also hear spiritually oriented persons speaking of a chakra opening as the process of becoming "self-realized" or "awakened" and that's another subject...that's a "grand opening!"

The good news is that you have the capability of boosting and balancing the chakras right in the palm of your hands! For example, visualize yourself waiting to be introduced. You are about to address 150 people...the butterflies are going wild. The trick is to get them to fly in formation! You can instantly soothe that feeling by merely *placing your hand over the third chakra,* just under your rib cage where your butterflies are, and intentionally sending some healing energy! Presto, your butterflies are flying in formation! If you are in a more private area and can add unruffling, so much the better!

In addition to placing a hand over the chakra (either above the body or actually touching the skin), some energize it by *moving the hand in a clockwise circle.* The most important ingredient is your intention to energize and balance the chakra.

Now, on to three ways to utilize the chakras in healing!

The Buddy System

There you are, wanting to relieve someone who's in pain and you have very little time. The "buddy system" is a shortcut version for spot treating an ailment quickly and effectively...faster than merely treating the problem area itself. By *energizing the nearest chakra* (major or minor) on either side of the problem, you have in a sense established a more vibrant circuitry in a localized area, which distinctly enhances the results.

Merely place your hands on the adjacent chakras to boost or energize them. Then move to the problem itself and do whatever intervention techniques you feel inclined to do. For example, if the problem is in the elbow, you would energize the shoulder and the wrist. If it were in the shoulder, energize the elbow and the throat or heart. (Don't get excited if you are confused as to where the *adjacent* chakra is, which one to use, or as in the case of a finger injury, you don't seem to find one on each side. Your intention will override the technique. Relax and flow with the process!) Once you've done the buddy system, you'll find the blockages are more apt to be in the mood to "get movin'." Any pain is inclined to leave faster.

The "Magnificent 7"

The second way to utilize the chakras is to use them for your own health maintenance and nurturing. I used to call on this technique when I felt a cold coming on or my energy level dropping. One day I noticed the fact that I was in a sense "disease oriented"...waiting for signs of disease or dysfunction before I bothered to enjoy some of what I so freely dished out to others on a regular basis. I wondered just what level of wellness I could sustain by giving myself a daily treatment.

I'm thrilled to tell you that since I have been doing the Magnificent 7 on a daily basis, I have never experienced even a cold or sore throat. I thought my energy level was excellent before, but I have now surpassed all previous personal levels of well-being. You might consider this your own personal wake-up call. Ten minutes is very little to ask for a body you so freely drive to the maximum!

The Magnificent 7 is done merely by placing your hands on each of the seven chakras individually for a couple of minutes each. If you do them in two's, you'll notice that you end up with one free hand at the crown. I place that hand anywhere else that seems to call to my attention.

Like everything else, you begin with the *triple awareness breath. I do the Magnificent 7 before rising each morning. It's a fabulous way to ready myself for the upcoming day. I arise with a sense of white light glowing in and around me and all major chakras humming in sync! And, as I put my foot on the floor, I say to myself, "Here We go!" (My spiritually connected "me"!)*

For years now, I've encouraged participants in my healing workshops to consider making a powerful decision. I ask them to declare that, for the next 21 days, (the time it takes to establish a new habit) they will begin each day by doing the Magnificent 7 technique on themselves. The feedback over the years has been absolutely astounding. People with insomnia are sleeping; those with mood swings are experiencing an even-ness in their emotions; travelers have used it successfully to prevent jet lag (myself included); those who found it most difficult to cope with each day are now coping more easily. Care to commit to 21 days beginning right now?

Sign here: _____!

Along with boosting and balancing my chakras, I use the time to clearly tell myself how much I appreciate "me." I thank all my "parts"...parts aren't just parts, you know! Life is about balance, learning to balance the *receiving* with the *giving*. The treatment itself sends an important message to me, about me. It says that *I am worthy*...worthy of the same wonderful attention I so freely pass out to others. I slip into a "best friend" role and the "two of me" trot off to greet the day! Perhaps the two of me will run into the "two of you" one of these days! We'll all smile knowingly!

Full Balancing Of Major And Minor Chakras

I melt just thinking about receiving this treatment. It is an extremely relaxing, energizing experience and ideal for a major overhaul. For those with serious illness, extremely low energy, or with generalized systemic problems (arthritis, leukemia, bone cancer, aids, etc.), it's best to call in the whole gang! Send some loving "light energy" to each chakra, major and minor (see Figure 7.11). What a wonderful treatment... I'm drifting off just thinking about it!

After intentionally boosting and balancing each major and minor chakra, you'll find a charmed moment in which everything else you do will be enhanced. It's a moment of receptivity in the body.

You may have noticed that the first major chakra is right over the pubic area. Actually, you are sitting on it! This is definitely an area to hold your hand above the body surface instead of on it! Did you understand that? Good!

I trust you will enjoy getting to know the chakras. They are as old as the earth itself, and yet offer you a superb new tool to use in healing!

To summarize, here is a list of the intervention techniques just covered:

- The Touch Itself...The Energy Flow

- Unruffling

- Massage

- Double Hand Boost

- The Laser

- Ultrasound

- Siphon

- Fluffing The Aura

- Reflexology...Painlessly

- The Back Package:

  –Massage

  –Thumb Walk

  –Hopi Indian Technique

  –Ultrasound

- Boosting And Balancing Chakras

- The Buddy System

- The "Magnificent 7"

- Boosting And Balancing Major And Minor Chakras

Chapter 8

Three Approaches To Healing

Got a minute? That's all you have? You'll find that along with the severity of the illness or dysfunction, and the physical environment you're working in, *time* is a major factor in determining which of the three approaches that you'll want to take in healing.

1. Sharing Energy: I say "sharing" because technically you are benefiting from the flow, too. This can be done merely to energize a tired co-worker or to boost someone's well-being. It involves the following:

    • Triple Awareness Breath

    • The Energy Flow

    • Disconnecting

2. This version is slightly longer and one in which you focus on a specific problem...headache, sore spot, sore throat, a burn, etc. You are addressing only one area of the body. It involves the following:

    • Triple Awareness Breath

    • Unruffle The Area

- The Buddy System (Energize The Two Adjacent Chakras)
- Intervention Techniques (Intuitive Work)
- Disconnect

3. This is the most lengthy version. It is a full body treatment that is used for people seriously ill or with systemic involvement (cancer, arthritis, chronic fatigue syndrome, fibromyalgia, severe burns, etc.). It can also be the ultimate in supportive health maintenance when absolutely nothing is wrong! I'd hop on your table in a flash to enjoy this kind of a treatment! Notice that due to the level of relaxation promoted in this version, grounding the healee is one of the important final steps.

- The Triple Awareness Breath
- The Scan (Optional)
- Unruffling The Area
- Boosting And Balancing Major And Minor Chakras
- Intervention Techniques
- Grounding The Healee
- Disconnecting

Chapter 9

The Tiny Clients... Infants!

Using healing touch on infants has been an absolute delight. As I mentioned earlier, one of the most reassuring experiences while working on premies (premature infants) has been that of the monitoring equipment confirming the effectiveness of the treatment.

Basically, the main difference in treating infants is the length of time of each treatment. Brief, intermittent sessions seem to work best, 30-60 seconds at a time when sending energy. Unruffling can be done effectively for much longer periods. It is great for fussy babies...calming them, relieving pain, and helping to reduce swelling or congestion.

With such a "tiny client" you can place one hand on the crown, the other on the soles of the feet and direct energy from head to foot. This can be used as a systemic boost, to boost and balance all chakras, and to generally accelerate all healing.

Ultrasound is great for pain, colic, digestive problems, respiratory problems, etc. Move clockwise above the area as if the body is the face of the clock. How do you spell relief? C-I-R-C-L-E-S!

You still use the six steps in a healing treatment for infants just as you do in treating adults. It's just shorter in duration and simpler!

Important points in working with newborns:

- *Talk* to him as you work. Acknowledge him and tell him what you are doing...or ways you'd like him to co-operate.
- *Slow down* when you move or touch him. Say "hello" with your hands before proceeding.
- When making physical contact, *land softly* or "feather-like." To break contact, even momentarily, *trail off* with your touch (rather than disconnecting abruptly). Land softly when you return.
- *Maintain touch* when at all possible so that he knows where you are. You are speaking with your every touch! One hand can reach for needed items while the other maintains contact, promoting his feeling of security.
- *Unruffle before and after procedures* such as changing diapers, etc.

The Touch Itself...
What Was That You Said?

Without saying a word your touch speaks volumes to the recipient. In it lies the key to reassure or alarm, to console or agitate, to gain a sense of trust or promote mistrust. In your touch lies your *intentionality*...directly responsible for your effectiveness as a healer. Being in touching professions (nursing and massage), I've long been aware of the power of touch. I've also been disappointed at how often its importance is minimized or forgotten amidst our fast-paced, high-tech society.

Granted, there are styles of healing in which no physical contact is made. In some states, this non-touching style is encouraged because of legal reasons. (You may want to find out whether you are "cleared for take off" in your area and can legally do hands-on-healing.) Often times the legality of doing hands-on-healing only pertains to those accepting payment for the healing treatment and there is no legal objection if the treatment is free.

I'm here to root for *touching* whenever possible. Having experienced both ways, I feel that even more can be enhanced with actual contact. I also feel strongly about the *style* of touch. Since I've worked with tiny premature babies, I thought perhaps allowing you to see it through a premie's eyes might make more of an impact.

Anne And Jeffery... A Tiny Love Story

[Jeffery] "Whoops...I'm here! And sooner than anyone expected! My parents are terrified...I can feel it in their trembling hands. The nurses are not happy with the readings on my monitoring equipment. I'm not a bit sure that I want to be here!

Everyone seems to be checking me over frequently...flipping me quickly from my back to my front, etc. It's a very efficient "flip" but makes my little head spin.

Ouch! Just when I was getting settled and thought I could take a 'breather,' someone whipped off my soft warm cover and pierced my foot with something terribly sharp! Something about a sample of my blood that they needed. My heart's pounding. It's difficult for me to breathe. I'm not going to take this quietly.

I must say the noise in here makes my little ears ache. Clanking of equipment, hubbub of chatter but no one talking to <u>me</u>, and on top of that...something called 'rock music' on a nearby radio. Not the station I'd choose! I need rock-a-bye music!

Once again two hands poke through the portholes of my isolette...this time I get the works. The blanket is yanked off, I'm manipulated this way and that...I'm flipped, suctioned, and repeatedly startled with an icy cold stethoscope hopping around on my chest and abdomen. Just when I think they've gone, in come two hands with more tasks. Finally, I am left to rest on my tummy. Up comes my soft warm blanket...my only friend! I'm given a gingerly pat on my bottom. I'm alone again. My heart is pounding! Is this the life that I have been preparing seven months for?

Whooa, I feel someone coming into my territory again...only this time the hands don't come in. Instead, I hear my name! I must be dreaming! A soft voice said, 'Hi, how ya doin' Jeffery? I'm Anne.' In come two loving hands, but neither touch me. Instead, one hand begins making a sweeping movement from my head to my toes. She does it two or three times...how soothing! Then her left hand lands ever so gently on the crown of my head...she cradles my head in her hand while gently saying 'hello' by way of a soft, thumb-stroke on my forehead.

Anne's right hand moves with feather softness to my back... I can feel its warmth right through the blanket. Anne says softly, 'Let's see what's goin' on with you, Jeffery!' (I love casual talk!) Her warm hand slowly removes my blanket. 'Let's turn you over, Jeffery,' Anne continues. This is amazing...suddenly I'm on my stomach! She did it ever so gently and in slow motion! Whew! I think I'm getting the hang of this!

While one hand is holding mine, once again Anne sweeps over me from head to foot a few times. I love it! She then slides one hand to my crown as her other hand lands gently on my feet. I can feel a warmth filling me from head to toe! It makes me tingle! She does this for about a minute.

Then I hear her say, 'I want to hear what's goin' on in this little chest of yours, Jeffery.' With one hand gently caressing my head, Anne listens to my chest. What a difference! She's using a WARM stethoscope! And instead of abruptly hopping from spot to spot, my new friend Anne gently and slowly *slides* it from spot to spot. Wow! What a difference when compared to my usual treatment!

While holding my hand, her other hand moves in a circular

motion above my chest...something about congestion in my lungs. I can already feel that it's easier to breathe.

Anne slowly pulls a soft blanket over me. After making one last sweep over my body (head to toe), I feel her reassuring hands trail away. It's not so bad here after all! Go ahead, check my monitor readings now!"

* * * * * * * * *

What's important for Jeffery is true for adults you work on as well. There's a real sense of trust that is built up when you know exactly where the healer is at all times and when the movement is slow and loving. Once you establish contact, try not to break it for any reason during the treatment. The main exception is during the Hopi Indian Technique in the third move when contact must be broken. Even then you can prepare the healee ahead of time so that the break is expected.

Say "hello" with your touch as you land feather softly. Say "goodbye" letting your fingers trail off. Let the part between your *hello* and *goodbye* convey the messages that: "You are safe...I care about your well-being...I'm here to help you...I have confidence in what I'm doing." It isn't about consuming more time than you normally would. (In fact, there's a very good chance that you'll be able to facilitate greater changes in a shorter amount of time since it entices the healee to join in the flow.) It's about being organized so that you can maintain contact as much as possible. It's about a healing style. (My fingers now trail away.)

Chapter 10

Healing Enhancers

The Importance Of Intention

You've certainly become familiar with intent by now! Your intention is woven in and out of the healing process in many ways. The key is to get in touch with as many facets as possible, becoming clearer and more purposeful as you do. Your lack of intention can mean that there is no particular benefit from the work, but an intention too specific can limit your work. There needs to be a happy medium in which you have a very clear intent to help or heal, but in a fairly broad way so that the energy can be allowed to be all that it can be! This will come with "intentional practice!"

Detaching Yourself From Outcomes

Although this has also been covered, it is one lesson that often has to be relearned. Healing isn't always "health," nor is it always in the form you'd expect. The energy always "works" on various levels, but you aren't in a position to judge the outcome. It may mean healing physical ailments, or it may mean resolving conflicts, healing relationships, or becoming more whole, balanced and at peace. So you see, you can experience a healing on some levels even if death is the ultimate outcome. Let go of the outcome! I said, "Drop it!" That's it! There goes another "outcome" falling to the ground...nice release!

Visualization

Since thought is energy and energy follows thought, what you visualize actually adds or detracts from the process on an energy level. As Geraldine used to say to Killer on the Flip Wilson Show, "What you see is what you get!" Whether you are working on someone with a known diagnosis, or you intuitively become aware of a possible tumor in the midst of a treatment, or perhaps you scan and perceive a specific disease condition, the important thing is to acknowledge the information and then visualize the health and wholeness in that same area.

Look at all negative findings as areas merely summoning your attention. Briefly notice what you are *not wanting* (e.g. blockage) and then immediately shift your attention to what you *are wanting!* Rather than flowing energy in order to "heal" the broken bone, celebrate the "healthy and whole" bone as you flow healing energy. Take your eyes off of what's wrong and find every creative way to celebrate the state of perfect health. Healing is about expanding into a greater truth rather than trying to rid the body of something. You might say that as a healer, you energetically entice others to open to the flow of Life Force that is their very nature. (See more about this in my book, *Sacred Choices: The gentle art of disarming a disease and reclaiming your Joy!*)

I find that visualization truly enhances this "cellular celebration" during my treatments. For example, if the healee is complaining of tremendous back pain, I immediately begin imagining him performing ballet movements (running, leaping, bending and stretching) in total comfort as I direct energy. If someone's shoulder is seized-up, I imagine them comfortably pitching softball; if they have respiratory difficulty, I imagine them taking in huge deep breaths of fresh mountain air. In other words, I focus my mind on the best example I can conjure up of the "opposite" and stay there during the rest of my treatment. I celebrate the body's magnificence!

In some instances, I silently affirm the message, "All is well!" (repeatedly) throughout the treatment. It's almost like a mantra or a chant that simultaneously gives me the vision of magnificence beneath my hands. It's like loving them into wholeness by energetically reminding them of who they really are.

We tend to give our power away to diseases, particularly cancer. Switching the focus away from cancer and to one in which you are merely restoring flow and balance diffuses the situation and allows you to reclaim your power. Visualization is the key. (If you are not a visual person or can't picture things, then just declare that the healee has a healthy body or that "All is well!") Declare or visualize light energy flowing freely from head to foot. What a marvelous picture! Get the Minolta!

Simplify

Don't get wrapped up in the details about what it is you are feeling during the treatment. It's really very simple. You allow light energy to flow through your hands to the healee, and it goes where it needs to go! With the proper intention, it is in exactly the right amount and duration. If you decide to scan, give up the need to label or diagnose. You merely note them as areas that call your attention.

Unlike the medical profession, success in healing does not depend upon a *diagnosis*. The focus is on *expanding health and wholeness* rather than on disease. One of my clients had periodic problems with severe back pain at the level of his heart. Heart disease had been ruled out on more than one occasion. His physician assured him that it was a back problem. I treated him during acute attacks with the back package. In minutes he was completely relieved and remained that way for months at a time. During his last acute attack, he saw his physician once more. On that visit it was finally discovered that it was his heart after all and was taken to surgery for a quadruple bi-pass the very next morning. My point is that it didn't matter what the diagnosis was...the energy went where it needed to go and brought prompt relief. It helped even when the actual problem was being missed on a medical basis and when I allowed the energy to go where it needed to go for the highest good. *Simplify!*

Unconditional Love

Have you ever heard of "unconditional love"? This is love—not when you get thinner, not after your acne clears up—but right now, before anything changes. It has nothing to do with loving any perceived imperfections in themselves or approving of outrageous behavior (yours, mine or theirs), or liking a disease, but rather of knowing a bigger truth. The truth is that there is a *greater you or authentic you* that is always "in there" on a deeper level—even when we temporarily have no sense of this magnificent "self." And, within each new day we have a renewed opportunity to make a powerful choice regarding our "selves" and others. We can choose to love who we really are—even before we can see it. We can choose to find things to focus on that delight us. We can choose to think thoughts that feel good. We can choose to gather the longest possible list of things we appreciate in life. And the pay-off? Whatever we focus our attention on in life, increases. It's the Law of Attraction. It's the precise reason we often hear life mantras of "the better it gets, the better it gets" or "the worse it gets, the worse it gets"!

So, what has your attention? Are you welcoming health... or at war with a disease? Are you appreciating, celebrating, and laughing uproariously... or, are you resenting, criticizing, worrying, doubting, fearing or feeling very right about someone else's wrong? The good news is that you don't have to "try" (for example) to stop worrying—you merely turn your focus to thoughts that feel better. Your emotions are your barometer... if what you are thinking feels good, your valve to well-being and health is wide open. But, if you are thinking thoughts that feel bad (no matter what the reason), you've just closed the valve to your well-being (financial abundance, good health, energy, healthy relationships, etc.).

So you can look at unconditional love as loving, just for the sake of loving—or feeling good, just for the sake of feeling good. Love is our nature. We are natural born lovers! This love can range from a feeling of peacefulness or well-being to outrageous joy. In either case, the critical shift is that, in that same instant, we have simultaneously opened to divine flow. (Read that again!) It means we are choosing to say "Yes!" to life rather than shouting "No!" to what we are not wanting. This has nothing to do with trying to paint black, white. Rather it has to do with expanding into what we would like rather than doing battle with what we find unacceptable. There is a profound difference in results. As we open to divine flow (spiritual connection), life works. Ever notice that when two people fall madly in love, all other areas of their life seem to be enhanced as well? Opportunities abound. Energy soars. We flourish. We thrive. We love!

Unconditional love—it's a daily game of finding a way (any way) to feel good. It's taking your attention off of what is and fixing your attention on how you would like it to be. This love is the very essence of the "light energy" itself... a flow of pure love. It's a choice. Ahhh, let the flow begin!

Expecting

Miracles are very normal. I noticed a unique correlation as I began experiencing more and more outward demonstrations of success. The more confidence I had in the healing energy, the more "demos" I saw. I was also comfortable with the times when nothing outward seemed to happen since this works on unseen levels as well. (Remember detaching yourself from the outcome?) Since energy follows thought, I realized that this *expectation* and *confidence* in the healing energy actually *intensifies the process*. It's worth your expectation! (And then your detachment!) It goes like this...Expect, then release! Very nice!

Energy Pillows

These pillows have brought tremendous comfort to literally hundreds of people. They are made with 100 percent cotton batting sold in some fabric stores. This unprocessed cotton has the ability to hold energy for months and even years. It offers some explanation of the therapeutic value we found in our stuffed teddy bears as kids. We were absolutely bonded with these stuffed little friends who were undoubtedly packed full of loving energy.

I have found that energy pillows can offer pain relief in everything from musculoskeletal problems, post-operative incisions, headaches and sinus problems, to babies with colic. I cut the cotton batting into eight by ten inch squares and slide it into a soft 100 percent cotton flannel pillowcase that I've made to cover it with. This gives you the opportunity to take off the case for laundering. For knee problems, I make a long pillow with ties on each end to hold it in place.

To energize a pillow, merely hold it between your hands for about five minutes while intentionally flooding it with healing energy. (In emergency situations in which I found myself rushing to the hospital to treat someone who was just injured, I energized it by holding it next to my body with one hand and driving with the other!) Placing it over a painful area can bring marvelous relief. I had one client who pitched for a softball team and had been suffering with a sore shoulder. (You must know how devastating that is to these men who take their team sports so seriously!) His shoulder cleared up promptly once he began sleeping with the energy pillow anchored on his shoulder. One day he called up in an absolute panic, his wife had accidentally sent the pillow through the laundry. (Cotton batting doesn't wash well at all!) I quickly made him another one. He won the game!

In summary, these seven things can enhance healing:

- Your Intention
- Detaching Yourself From Outcomes
- Visualizing
- Simplifying
- Unconditional Love
- Expecting...
- Energy Pillows

Chapter 11

A Quick Reference For Specific Problems

These are merely ideas to get you started. I am assuming that you will include your own *intuitive* ideas as well.

- **Abdominal Cramps, Stomach Distress, Nausea, Colic:** Unruffle. Move in a clockwise circle over the stomach or abdomen. On abdominal work, make circles large enough in diameter to include entire abdomen.

- **Angina:** Unruffle. Double hand boost over the heart. Include prescribed medication as needed.

- **Back Problems:** Unruffle. Energize chakras in ankles, knees and hips. Utilize the techniques in the back package.

- **Broken Bones:** Works right through casts. Unruffle. The buddy system technique. Ultrasound technique. Energy pillow.

- **Burns:** Unruffle, unruffle, unruffle!

- **Emotional Crisis:** Unruffle. Boost and balance all chakras. Shorter version: energize third and fourth chakras (solar plexus and heart chakras).

- **Fatigue, Exhaustion:** Unruffle. Boost and balance major and minor chakras. Shorter version: send energy through the shoulders.

- **Fussy Babies:** Unruffle.

- **Headaches:** Unruffle. Energize the throat and crown chakras. Ultrasound.

- **Injuries:** The quicker you intervene, the better. Unruffle. The buddy system technique or boost and balance all chakras, depending on the severity. Ultrasound injured area. Remember to also include appropriate emergency first aid measures as well.

- **Menstrual Cramps:** Unruffle. Boost first and second chakras. Double hand boost technique. Ultrasound technique. Can also place one hand on the coccyx (tail bone), the other over the lower abdomen, and allow the energy to flow between the two.

- **Sore Muscles Or Painful Spot:** Unruffle. Double hand boost technique on the area. Ultrasound technique.

- **Reflexology Points Or Acupressure Points:** Unruffle the point. Double hand boost technique. Ultrasound. Recheck the point and repeat process as needed.

- **Sinus Problems, Tooth Aches, Ear Aches, Eye Problems:** Unruffle. Boost throat and crown chakras. Double hand boost technique. Ultrasound.

- **Swelling (Edema):** Unruffle. The buddy system technique, then lots of unruffling.

Chapter 12

𝒟elightful 𝒟emos

A great part of the success in hands-on-healing is in *remembering to use it!* We have so many well-programmed internal cassettes that spring us into action for specific problems. Someone says, "Looks like Strep Throat," and we're out the door to get a throat culture and antibiotics without hesitation—but haven't we forgotten something? We could also have done some healing!

I am not sharing the following demos to convince you of the effectiveness of this work, but merely to inspire you. Seeing how healing can be blended into everyday life situations may mean that an inner light bulb will flip on when you see a similar circumstance and you'll be brave enough to try!

Post-Operative

Doug, a neighbor of mine, was in a serious automobile accident. Four vertebrae were injured, two of them crushed. I first saw him the day after his surgery in which metal rods were inserted into his spine. Doug was absolutely miserable. Not only was he in pain from his back, but his abdomen was very distended (swollen) with gas, due to the temporary lack of bowel function. Unrelieved by any of the pain medications given, he was almost constantly in motion (slow motion) from side to side attempting to gain some level of comfort.

After a few questions and an assessment of the situation, I began working on his feet. This seemed appropriate for several reasons. First of all, as yet, I had no idea whether Doug was open to hands-on-healing. Secondly, so much can be enhanced through the reflex points in the feet. Doug was not only delighted that the massage felt wonderful, but also that he could feel his feet. (He had been told prior to the surgery that there was a surgical risk of paralysis from the waist down.)

As we talked a little more, Doug seemed open to what I described as "some very gentle and relaxing work that could help relieve pain." I unruffled him and began carefully placing my hands on his back and switching to his abdomen as he rolled back and forth. I also used the ultrasound technique on his abdomen.

Just after I initially placed my hands on his back, he exclaimed to his wife almost tearfully, "Jean, I can feel that going clear down in my toes!" By then I had no doubt that I could openly proceed with whatever felt appropriate. (Let the fun begin!)

I worked for about 45 minutes doing more of the techniques already described as well as boosting and balancing his chakras, and intuitive work. In addition, I gave him his very own energy pillow which became his constant companion. When I left, Doug was lying still and was comfortable for the first time. His bowels began to function that afternoon and the distension left in his abdomen.

Doug was doing extremely well when I returned the next morning to give him another treatment. From the time of the very first treatment, Doug never took nor needed another pain medication during the remainder of his hospitalization. He went home three days after I initially saw him. I continued to treat him regularly, using the Hopi Indian Technique and added massage as his back permitted. He continued to show an accelerated rate of healing during his entire recovery period.

* * * * * *

Another friend of mine, Phyl, had major abdominal surgery. Since family members frequently are allowed to see the patient before I can, I often put them to work as well. I give them instructions on how to send energy to the chakras while holding the patient's feet.

As previously mentioned, chakras tend to block due to the insult of the surgery. The sooner they re-open and stay that way, the faster the patient gets all "systems" working and gets well. (We all know what systems those nurses are interested in, huh!)

Phyl's husband, Bob, was glad to participate. (This is a great way to counteract the feeling of helplessness often experienced when a loved one goes to surgery. They love having something to do that can be beneficial.) I also taught Phyl how to do the Magnificent 7 technique and gave her an energy pillow. Bob eagerly did his part, as did Phyl. When I saw her for the first time the day after surgery she was looking radiant. As I unruffled her, and boosted and balanced her chakras, she excitedly recounted the previous day's experience. Upon returning to her room from surgery, she persuaded a reluctant nurse to let her sit up, then dangle her legs off the side of the bed, then to walk to the nurse's station and back. Phyl remained totally comfortable without any pain medication and spent the rest of her two-day stay trying to convince the staff that she was not being a martyr...she was just plain fine!

Strokes

Last summer, I picked up my 66-year old neighbor Charlie from the airport who had just returned from a vacation in New York. As we stopped to have lunch on the way home, he began complaining of feeling very strange. Although he knew where he was and that he had just returned from New York, he could not remember his address or telephone number (of the past 12 years). At his insistence, I drove him home rather than to a doctor. I checked his blood pressure, which was normal, but his symptoms continued. He was emphatic about not seeking medical attention. Reluctantly, I ran to keep a previous appointment but checked with him periodically by phone. When I returned a few hours later there had been no improvement. I then gave him a treatment, including unruffling, boosting and balancing his major chakras, and intuitive work around his head. In minutes his memory was totally back.

Although Charlie's symptoms were certainly indicative of a light stroke, it remains a good example to remember. Hands-on-healing provides the perfect thing to do when there's nothing else to do. In more serious cases, if time permits, it can be added to the treatment given during an ambulance ride or while waiting for help to arrive.

Eye Injuries

Well now, there's my dog, Buttercup, who never can seem to keep her nose out of the cat's reach. She loves to antagonize! A few years ago, she did it one too many times and received a frightening eye injury with old Ms.'s right hook! At 6 a.m. one Saturday morning as I was sorting laundry, Buttercup casually strolled into the room. I reached down to pet her and nearly fainted at what I saw. She had blood all over the side of her face and looked as if she had lost her eye. It would be a couple of hours before I could get her in to see my veterinarian. In the meantime, I held my hands over her eye every chance I got. Later, when she was examined by my veterinarian, he treated her by temporarily sewing her eye lid shut. He told me that the prognosis for her eye was guarded and that she might lose the sight in that eye. I continued to give her treatments several times a day. A week later, to the amazement of the vet, her eye had been saved. During that week I had treated her regularly with unruffling, the double hand boost technique, and ultrasound.

Although her eye was saved, she was left with a large white scar near the center of it. My veterinarian asked me if I'd like him to surgically remove the scar. I declined. During the few weeks that followed, I continued to treat Buttercup regularly. She ended up with two beautiful eyes and absolutely no trace whatsoever of the injury or the scar!

Cancer

Hands-on-healing is a wonderful way to deal with cancer. For those having chemotherapy, regular healing treatments can actively diminish or eliminate side effects. This includes hair loss. At a time when the person is often feeling victimized and helpless, being taught simple ways to draw in healing is a major comfort. The Magnificent 7 technique can provide tremendous support on a daily basis.

A few years ago, I had a 30-year old client who had been operated on for a malignant brain tumor. The doctors were unable to remove all of it. One day, she came to me extremely depressed and terribly weak. She stated that her "white count" (white cells in the blood) was so low that they were unable to give her more chemotherapy. To top that off, her one eye was bulging which was causing her vision to blur, and the four-month old incision at the back of her head was hurting. She complained of a feeling of pressure in her head.

This was the first time she had agreed to let me use healing techniques on her. I boosted and balanced her chakras and did some intuitive work around her head. I used the ultrasound technique around her incision. An hour later she got off my table excitedly describing all the changes that had occurred. Her energy was fully revitalized, all pressure in her head had ceased, and her eye had returned to normal. A CAT scan test two days later revealed that the tumor had decreased to a third of its previous size!

Angina

They're all over Florida—senior citizens who come here to enjoy retirement, only to develop heart problems that drastically dampen much of their fun and keep them fearful about enjoying physical activities. Many have exhausted potential medical and surgical possibilities and find themselves saddled with the realization that their only option is to just learn to live within their limitations and stay close to home.

People with cardiac problems have their hands full trying not to complicate the situation with anxiety. For these people, nighttime can feel horribly long when twinges and worrisome chest pains once again surface. Spouses and loved ones can also feel a real sense of helplessness. A good day is often one in which nothing worse happens. Self-esteem and identity quickly fade when people can't be who they really are. This is certainly not what they had planned! The good news is that this is where healing energy can play a tremendous role for everyone concerned.

I have had a number of clients who were experiencing bouts of angina (pain often radiating down the left arm due to lack of oxygen to the heart muscle). Unruffling the chest area and sending healing energy to the heart has proven to be extremely beneficial in controlling the symptoms. Some people have a vague sense of *impending angina* that serves to warn them before angina actually appears. Placing their own hand over their heart and intentionally sending energy is often all it takes to make it disappear. For times when angina actually surfaces, energy work can be done right along with taking prescribed medications. It's very common to find that less medication is needed and that these people find that the pain subsides more easily. The neat thing is that the spouse can help with the treatment, too—or it can be administered by the person himself.

Many have found that doing the Magnificent 7 treatment on a daily basis greatly lessens the angina attacks. Hands-on-healing...perfect for those anxious days and nights! It's something to do during those times you previously thought nothing could be done!

Premature Infants

Jeffery was born 12 weeks prematurely, weighing only two and a half pounds. His mother, Linda, immediately got to work creating a healing environment. She encouraged hospital staff and family members to visualize Jeffery surrounded in white light. On every visit, Linda unruffled Jeffery and directed energy for short periods. She shared healing ideas with the staff and encouraged them to touch him "intentionally" as well.

Linda pumped her breasts and made frequent trips to the hospital to deliver breast milk for Jeffery's feedings. With a husband and three other children at home, life was definitely a challenge. Running on very little sleep, she was literally sustained by meditating twice a day and drawing in healing energy.

Jeffery did extremely well. You may already be aware that being premature often means several years before the child catches up with others who were born full-term. At only 10 months of age, Jeffery's doctor found that there was *absolutely no lag in his cognitive skills*. He was just like any normal ten-month old. You may have noticed that premature babies often have narrow odd-shaped heads for some time. Jeffery's head was well shaped from the first few days.

Jeffery and Linda made such an impact on the hospital staff and nursery that they literally paved the way for healing techniques. They were instrumental in helping to set up hands-on-healing training programs within the neonatal unit. They both remain an inspiration to those of us who saw this beautiful story unfold.

Broken Bones

A friend of mine, Marge, fell while riding her bike and injured her wrist. Her doctor diagnosed it as a fracture and put her wrist in a splint. Once the swelling was down, he planned to put it in a cast.

Marge agreed to try a treatment just to see what it would do. Her hand was slightly blue in appearance and very swollen. It resembled the look of a blue glove filled with water. She was in pain. Leaving it in the splint, I utilized unruffling, the buddy system, ultrasound, and the double hand boost technique. Magically, during the treatment, a great deal of the swelling went down and her pain was relieved. Marge continued to send energy to her wrist each day. Two days later her doctor shook his hand and told her that it was doing so well there was no need to cast it.

Sunburn

When our son, Linc, was 16 years old, he came home with a terrible sunburn. That was during the same period when he thought my healing techniques were ridiculous. After suffering for several hours with chills and discomfort, he became motivated to let me do my "thing." I decided it was the perfect opportunity to do just half of his sunburn. I repeatedly unruffled only the right side of his body. The next day, the right side was great. The left side was sore and had blisters. He said it was because he had burned the other side more! Ahhh, to be 16 years old again and know everything! (P.S. At 18 years of age he has come full circle and lets me work on him any time.)

Plants

When we were moving from Denver to Orlando, Florida, the man from the moving company advised me not to take my plants. He said, "Lady, it takes me five days to get there. The truck is not insulated and the boxed plants will have to endure over 100 degree temperatures." I smiled at him and told him I still wanted them to go.

They sealed the plants in boxes, leaving them in the house that night so that they would be loaded last. I talked to them all (in their boxes), telling them where they were going and that they would love it. I energized each plant. Not only did they make it, but they came out of the boxes looking as if they had never traveled—even my "fussy ficus" tree!

Animals

I love working on animals. In the past I've donated my time to the Humane Society after gaining permission to do healing on the animals there.

A friend of mine had an Arabian horse that had been limping around with an arthritic knee. I leaped at the opportunity to work on him. For 20-30 minutes I worked on his knee, using unruffling, ultrasound and the double hand boost, and praying he wouldn't step on me! His knee has been fine every since!

Another animal client was a 13-year old shepherd dog with terrible arthritis. She couldn't even get her head down to her water bowl at times. I worked on her about every three months.

Generally, I used a lot of unruffling and ultrasound on her joints. Each time she would magically transform into a freely moving, playful, energetic dog!

I continue to donate my time to anyone who has an animal in need of healing. I see the animal once and teach the owner how to continue with healing techniques on a regular basis. The phone calls and notes I receive regarding success stories continue to be a delight. The pet owners are thrilled with their new-found techniques for health, and so glad they are able to enhance the lives of the pets they adore!

Chapter 13

Living In Healing Ways

We see it over and over in nursing. A patient is given the sobering news that he has a serious disease. Frequently, it leaves him quickly scanning his life to see how it all happened. He is filled with remorse. "If only I would have..." or "I should have..." (Ever hear of the saying, "I shall not *should* on myself today?")

In most cases, it isn't just one thing that promoted the illness. By the same token, there isn't just one path to the cure. Hands-on-healing is merely part of the answer. It is not meant to be used in place of sound medical treatment, but as a complement to it. There are many ways to promote optimum health on a daily basis.

Health is about balance. We may be paying attention to the body but boldly ignoring the emotional or spiritual self. We often drive our bodies rather than honor them. The difference can be as subtle as exercising because we have to, or exercising because we like taking excellent care of our bodies and we're worth it! Your body knows the difference. All the health food and exercise in the world can't make up for carrying around hate, resentment, and lack of forgiveness. On the other hand, when there is a deep level of love and forgiveness for yourself and others, it automatically makes you inclined to take loving care of the physical body.

Minor illnesses that we get along the way are marvelous stretches of "down time" or "time-outs" in life. Perfect opportunities that we create in order to return to balance. This "stretch" most often signals that we've come up short on the receiving end. You might look at it as your body's way of requesting, and hopefully getting, your undivided attention for an exceptionally good cause—your personal well-being.

Even though it is normally quite energizing to give a healing treatment, there is a definite need to learn when to say "no." For example, the process of doing a healing provides a nice pick-me-up when you are slightly fatigued. However, there is a point that you will learn to identify within your own body when you need to focus the healing energy on you and postpone the work on others. If you're not careful, your ego will have you convinced that others can't make it without you. It's a nice lesson to see that you said "no" and everyone managed just fine.

In terms of health and disease, let's take a look at where we are *participating* with each.

Self-Talk = Cell Talk!

(Take One...and...Action!) The scene is 6:00 a.m. Monday morning after a weekend of over-indulging...your alarm sounds...you stumble to the bathroom and gaze into the mirror in a stupor as the "unforgiving" fluorescent light goes on. Squinting at the familiar face staring back, you feel the painfully candid zing of your constant companion...your ever-present internal critic. You know, the one you take so seriously! The negative verbiage rolls as you take in a "close-up" shot...more bags, more sags...the "aging" fairy was sprinkling you in your sleep again! You accept what you consider to be the truth about you. It's a wrap. More accurately, *it's a rap!*

How's your "self-talk" lately? You know, the statements you feel so free to spew at yourself day in and day out...critiquing and judging your every move! All of us feel so comfortable saying the most outrageous things to ourselves. We think it's okay because we're only talking to ourselves, and no one's listening anyway. Surprise! On a cellular level, you are listening to every thought.

I like to picture the human cell as a cute little circle with two eyes and two ears. What cells do best is obediently respond to your thoughts (self-talk) and what you are visualizing. Since they don't have a mouth, they don't give us any "back-talk." They just respond. We often give them conflicting messages so they respond to what you think about the most.

Probably the best illustration of cellular response to thought is one previously mentioned (and worth repeating) regarding people with split personalities. Their bodies listen to their thoughts, and as the personalities shift, the new thoughts and belief system paired with that personality immediately choreograph totally different versions of the "self" *within the exact same body*. Suddenly, the pancreas stops working or a cigarette burn disappears. When the previous personality returns, the pancreas fires right up again working just fine, and the burn reappears.

Granted, for most of us our changes are slower and much more subtle, but we are always moving in the direction of our thoughts. Many times it can even be seen in the way people tend to carry themselves. For example, it's very common to find rounded or bent shoulders in someone who feels emotionally unsupported in life and feels they carry a weight on their shoulders daily. The body never argues! Take a quick look to see what statement your body is making right now. Scan your body, your posture, and your apparent level of health. Are you sitting in a slump with your ribs compressing your liver? Are you holding that stomach in or just letting it all hang out? Really! Are you experiencing optimum health or are you barely staying afloat... an accident waiting to happen?

There you are in your daily movie, "On the Road to Enough." (No, this is not one of Bob Hope's road films!) Your lines are very simple but repetitive.

- "I'm not good enough."

- "I'm not tall (or short) enough."

- "I'm not thin enough."

- "I'm not pretty (or handsome) enough."

- "I'm not rich enough."

- "I'm not tan enough."

- "I'm not smart enough."

...And the bottom line for most of us is: "I'M NOT ENOUGH!"

With your lines extremely well-rehearsed, you then point yourself toward a new goal while saying "Now, get out there and be all you can be!" (Right!) Then you wonder why you can't seem to be as perfect as you'd like to be.

But on to the good news. Thoughts can be changed. You can put in a new software program about yourself any time you choose...one that contains positive affirmations about *who* and *what* you are. It's good to state everything in the present tense as if it has already happened. For example, "I now find it very easy to be flexible and flowing with life." Steer clear of phrases like "going to" since it essentially refers to things in the future—things that will happen in the future which tend to keep it out of reach for this moment.

Years ago, I stumbled across a book by Louise Hay entitled *Heal Your Body*. I quickly noticed that a number of her philosophies seemed to step right along with my own. Her book contains a list of bodily symptoms and diseases. Each physical symptom on the list is followed by a probable cause and a healing affirmation, or a new thought pattern. I browsed through it looking up problems I had noted in friends and clients, etc. The issue she listed for each seemed to be right on target. I was fascinated. I gingerly looked up "knees" since I had been plagued with bad knees for years. I was totally taken aback. It said something about having a stubborn ego and pride, and not being flexible. I stiffened. I thought to myself (with jaw clenched), "I *am* flexible. I am one of the most flexible people I know!" I seriously believed that. As time went on, I was eventually able to see that I did have *areas* of inflexibility.

The knees kept getting worse. I grew to be all arm power when going down stairs...a grip of death on the hand railing. Handicap restrooms with the bars on either side of the wall had wonderful appeal. Eventually arthroscopic surgery on one knee revealed that the cartilage was missing in most of the joint. I was finally ready to actively address a new thought pattern. I began to proclaim my flexibility in life and my ability to flow and bend with ease. I told my knees how flexible and flowing they were and that they served me well. With the last statement, I doubled over in laughter. It seemed so far from what I saw as the reality! Then I got so that I could say it without laughing. After a while, I got so that I could pour myself into the affirmation with total sincerity. I also affirmed my love not only for my knees, but for all of me.

Well, here I am years later, the proud owner of two great knees. If you have a minute, I'll show you how I can go down stairs without my previous grip of death on the railing. I easily sit on the floor cross-legged. Even more fascinating to me is the fact that I can then get up and walk away in total comfort! I continue to affirm that I am flexible and flowing with life. My knees are smiling as I write this...they love this story. (Have you ever seen knees smile?)

Some time back, I had the occasion to look up another subject in Louise Hay's book. The problem was listed as anger. Quickly, I thought, "Louise, Louise, Louise...you're off the mark on this one. I'm not angry at anyone!" Two days later it hit me. I had been looking "out there" for where I might be focusing anger. It was much closer to home. I was angry at me. I tend to be very visual and see goals I want to accomplish. Before I can even reach the goal, I see more to accomplish and better ways to do it and create a new goal. In other words, I never arrive! I was beating myself up for not being perfect enough, and never acknowledging my accomplishments. Even when others would rave about all I had done, I couldn't take it in. I knew that it wasn't perfect enough. The new and wiser me began praising myself for my accomplishments. I began "praising in the present"...without looking back or forward to greater or lesser things. I began actively and consistently forgiving myself for everything. Over a period of time, the condition consistently improved.

So you see, the negative emotion or issue can be an "inside job." The saying, "What goes around, comes around," not only applies to life "out there," but to the critical circle of how you are treating you.

Louise Hay doesn't necessarily have the last word as to what the problem is but her list provides a great place to start. Consider it *possibility thinking*...that maybe, just maybe this could be true. You know, be flexible and flowing about it all. Ahem! Then get busy with your new self-talk.

This is a grand beginning on the road to creating the new you. The one you really want to be! The one you'll gradually discover isn't so bad after all and who grows easier to love everyday. It's as simple as changing the message. Make a list of affirmations for yourself. Think them, write them, and speak them as often as possible. Record your affirmations on tape and play it as often as you can even if you aren't consciously listening to it. Blend the affirmations into as much of your day as possible. I personally love to talk out loud to myself in the car. It seems like a safe place to pour myself into exuberant self-talk that I'd be too self-conscious to do other places. Try it for yourself! Pour yourself into your self-talk with the conviction and enthusiasm you show to others when you're supporting them.

You'll be amazed at how much more energy you have when you don't have the "Negative Nellie" hanging on you all the time. Life will seem lighter. Someday along the way, you'll notice that the bottom line in your daily movie is no longer "I'm not good enough." Instead you smile as you lovingly and passionately belt out, "I <u>am</u>!"

Gentle Care And Feeding Of The Psychological You!

Although many are focused on personal growth these days, it's understandable that many others would rather bury themselves in work, outer-oriented tasks, alcohol, or drugs than peek inward. Who wants to get to know themselves better if they think that all that's "in there" is a painful abundance of imperfection? Drugs and alcohol get the negative self-talk to stop, and provide very temporary internal peace. Another misguided version is the over-achiever, the workaholic. Over a period of time the over-achiever identifies so much with his job and title that he often becomes the title. He thinks *that's who he really is.* Remove his career entirely and he may feel that he ceases to exist. This can cause a severe emotional crisis when a health condition brings a career to a permanent halt. Meanwhile, his inner self waits patiently to be acknowledged, loved, and understood.

What if you constantly poured that kind of script into a child? What kind of self-esteem would you expect that child to have? Think of that same child filled with loving support...a child who hears things like "I love you just the way you are...You can never lose my love...I'm always here for you...I understand...You can do it."

The truth is that psychologically all of us do have a "child self" right inside, one that never grows up. Part of living in healing ways is to *intentionally say the type of supportive things to ourselves (inner child included) that we would freely dish out to support anyone we loved.* Many of us run around looking for someone who understands us. Have you ever thought of telling yourself that "you understand"? Or, during a stressful situation, how about telling yourself, "Now, take it easy. You're doing just fine." In other words, be your own best friend wherever you go!

(Replay with a twist.) The scene is 6:00 a.m. Monday morning after a weekend of over-indulging...your alarm sounds...you stumble into the bathroom and look into the mirror as the unforgiving fluorescent light goes on...(smiling lovingly) you wink and wave! (Congratulations, you just passed a semester final in *Living in Healing Ways 101!)*

Gentle Care And Feeding Of The Emotional You!

You just did it again. When will you ever learn to keep your mouth shut? Your words hurt someone you care deeply about. You're filled to the brim with remorse and *guilt.* (Ahh yes, give the gift that keeps on giving, give guilt!)

In his album titled *Secrets of the Universe,* Wayne Dyer talks about a marvelous imaginary planet. Anytime the people there encounter guilt, they can opt to go into "rewind" and relive that portion differently!

But, here we are, playing out our reality on planet earth. We become so accustomed to carrying around guilt, resentments, anger, self-criticism, emotional pain, etc., that this is what we actually identify with as being normal. While those negative emotions take their toll on our bodies, the good news is that the reverse is also true. As Bernie Siegel (author of *Love, Medicine, and Miracles*) puts it, there are "physiological consequences of love, hope, joy, and optimism." Your body thrives on these kinds of consequences!

Two magical standard ingredients help in every situation. They are love and forgiveness. The first place to begin is right inside you, loving and forgiving <u>you</u>. The delight is that as you change, everyone benefits. As you begin to love yourself more, you find an increased capacity to love everything and everyone. You feel less need to control and consequently, you become more flexible. You become less fearful because you feel supported internally. You find more joy in life itself because you are perceiving it from a loving viewpoint.

So you think it sounds like a good idea, but you find many things about yourself so unlovable? After all, you have been keeping a detailed record, updated to the previous minute that just passed, of all your imperfections and places you haven't measured up! And, you feel that if people saw this long list of imperfections, no one would like you! It's good that you can at least fool others. Or, perhaps you feel that if you loved and accepted yourself with all your faults that you would never be motivated to improve. Is that what's bothering you?

Loving yourself unconditionally is the grandest foundation to base all change on. You'll find all personal growth much easier when coupled with forgiveness and love. It's as easy as changing your internal messages. It's as easy as taking on new self-talk filled with love and forgiveness. As you gain increased success with that single focus, your ability to forgive and love others will automatically follow. The wheels will be set in motion to attract healthier and happier relationships.

* * * * * *

You just did it again. You just put your foot in your mouth. It was quite a disappointment because your life is changing in very positive ways, and you seem to go for longer periods of time using your feet for transportation purposes only. This time the "new you" instantly springs into action. Along with any appropriate adjustment you can make with whoever received your inappropriate remark, you simultaneously relay an internal supportive message of forgiveness and unconditional love for yourself. It beats your previous self-flogging style, hands down. As soon as you can, you follow up by placing your hand over your solar plexus (the area right under your ribs in which you normally feel the blow to your self-esteem) and send some healing energy to your wound. There's nothing like having a compassionate and supportive "internal" best friend!

Your Back Speaks...

"Now, you want me to do what?"

You reply, "I just want you to twist, contort, and lean at a right angle for an hour or so! I'm sure you won't mind because it's for a good cause. You know, anything to help others!"

While some are campaigning to "Save The Whales," I'm here on official business to "Save The Backs!" There are many ways to do hands-on-healing and *take good care of your own back* at the same time. Massage tables are ideal. Since most people don't have them, other spots provide ideal substitutions. For example, a dining room table, kitchen counter (especially a three-sided-island counter), picnic table, etc. (You probably thought I'd include the hood of the family car or the roof of the tool shed!)

A sheet or a pad placed under the healee can be used to pull them closer to you as you work from each side. The closer you are to them, the less strain on your back. Try to keep your knees slightly flexed rather than locked. Adjust your height by moving your feet farther apart or switching from shoes to bare feet.

Many healers work with the healee in a chair. They have them sit sideways, with the back of the chair at either side. This gives them the opportunity to reach most of the body of the healee. In this position, it's even more important to bend the knees instead of stooping over. Kneeling is also appropriate. Do your knees the favor of providing a pillow to kneel on!

Laying your hands right on the healee (lightly) is easier on your back than holding your hands in the air for lengthy periods of time. When doing work on a table, moving to the opposite side is often more comfortable than reaching across. You may discover ways in which you can curl your fingers over and under the opposite limb and actually lean slightly on your knuckles at the same time. If you notice your own back is beginning to ache, take in a deep breath and intentionally let go of the tension in that area. The bottom line is to maintain a body awareness as you work. Your back says "thank you!"

You're excited about healing, you want to share it...but how?

I find that the easiest way to share healing with those who have never experienced it is with a lot of enthusiasm and openness to "just see if it can help." Remember, you can never promise what the outcome will be. In a sense, both of you, the healer and the healee, stand back and watch. The more the healee has tried other avenues unsuccessfully, the more he or she tends to be open to this simple, natural process. In fact, my ears perk up and my palms warm in just hearing the words, "They say nothing more can be done!"

The healee's spiritual or religious orientation is a major consideration in offering a healing treatment. There are some religions that take a dim view of the very process that you and I cherish. Some look at it as one that can only be done by people chosen by God. The very process that enhances one person can make those of a different orientation feel vulnerable and at risk. Since the only job the healee has in order to benefit is to allow the process, there is no way any change can take place in someone who feels at risk, and who is inadvertently blocking the process.

For those who have never received a healing treatment before but are willing to experience one, it helps to explain it in very natural ways. To anyone with an interest in gardening, I explain that the energy is for them like sunshine is to a plant. For those mechanically inclined, I speak of it as similar to "jump starting" a car. Boosting and balancing chakras can be likened to a tune-up. For those spiritually oriented and who identify with the divine energy, I describe the healing light that is filling them during the process. Some are familiar with chakras and I explain the use of energy to boost and balance them. Younger people who can identify with the movie *Star Wars* respond to the description of the energy as being "life force" and resonate to the expression, "May the Force be with you." Small children often respond well when perceiving it as receiving love. Your touch speaks loudest of all.

Listen closely for word cues in conversation. As you are gently pursuing philosophies, you'll often be able to pick up key words as to how open the person is to healing. Many have been involved in meditation, yoga, acupuncture, imagery, etc. For anyone who has experienced acupuncture or knows of it, you can relate the energy flow as being quite similar. You are sending the energy along similar pathways without the use of needles. The goal is similar in both cases. It is to re-establish flow and balance.

I describe the Hopi Indian Technique to clients as a marvelously gentle technique that gets the energy flowing in the back, and consequently promotes health. In nearly every case, people seem to be quite comfortable with the idea and feel that it is a very special technique to receive. They tend to love Indians!

For those receiving the ultrasound technique, I tell them that I'm moving my fingers around in a circle just above the area being treated. I describe the energy from my fingers as sweeping through even the deepest tissue, hastening the release of pain. Frequently, I'll have the healee choose a number from one to ten that corresponds to the pain being felt before the treatment has begun (ten being the greatest discomfort). It doesn't matter what the number is. I'm looking for a lower number each time I have him re-assess the discomfort. This normally works so well that the decreased pain speaks for itself. People seem to love the ultrasound technique!

Delegating Responsibility

Nice job! You were able to facilitate marvelous changes in the healee. But don't stop there! It's time to show him how HE can participate in his own wellness. The degree of his participation depends somewhat on where he stands in his awareness and belief system. Depending upon the comfort level of the client, I teach him to do the triple awareness breath, the unruffling technique, and the Magnificent 7 technique. Many leave with books to read, meditative tapes to listen to regularly, and even a song to sing twice a day entitled, "I love Myself The Way I Am," by Jai Josefs. (It's just like taking a very important medicine twice a day, only this medicine is in the form of a song!) I have them focus on ways to love themselves more and dole out little assignments to complete by the next week. I gently urge thoughtful, healthy eating and breathing, and encourage them to drink water. I teach them how to live in healing ways *without* me.

Healing In The Work Place

Many of us work in highly negative work places. Hospitals are no exception. Filling and surrounding yourself with white light before you arrive is a great way to decrease your vulnerability. Beginning the day with the Magnificent 7 technique for self-balancing and nurturing is also ideal. Surround your co-workers in white light as well. Many have found that they also feel better if they disconnect from the work environment with the step used for "termination" (a sweep of the hand down the front of the body) as they leave for the day.

You can also mentally clear out your work area by imagining a spinning ball of white light in the center of the room that continues to expand until it has pushed through every wall, ceiling, and floor. You may want to visually project filling the area back up with a certain color to promote the kind of environment you'd like. Although the same color can be used for varying effects, it again ties in with your intent. For example:

- Blue = calming or cooling

- Green = healing

- Pink = love

- Yellow = intellectual stimulation

You may want to send more than one color!

The unruffling technique is ideal for days in which nothing seems to be working or flowing. Take a break, take a breath, and unruffle!

So, you've arrived at your work place, the mall, or the supermarket, and you feel your energy level taking a rapid dive? You forgot to use the white light beforehand? An easy way to instantly stop the energy drain is just to place your hand on your third chakra (the solar plexus just under your rib cage). Then take in the triple awareness breath and send energy right back into yourself. Nice fueling, huh!

Nurses

You have charmed opportunities to intertwine healing techniques in with your care. If you're working in the Recovery Room, you can do a shortcut version of boosting and balancing chakras by holding the patient's feet (or placing your hands near them) and sending energy right up the body for a minute or so. The chakras that were blocked due to the insult of the surgery will be enhanced. The patient's body functions (peristalsis, urination, defecation) will return to normal much more quickly. If unruffling can be included, so much the better.

Energy can be sent to several major chakras when you are listening with a stethoscope to the chest and abdomen. Merely slide the diaphragm on the stethoscope between two fingers and let your open palm "linger" a bit as you listen. Let the energy flow through your palm at the same time.

For cramping or abdominal distension (providing that the patient is open to this process), use ultrasound. Move over the abdomen in large clockwise circles (as if the abdomen is the face of the clock).

For burns, unruffle, unruffle, unruffle! Before starting intravenous drips, unruffle the site before you begin. When removing intravenous needles, unruffle the site after you withdraw the needle or catheter to help close the puncture site.

Massage Therapists

You'll get faster results with deep tissue work if you first use healing energy on the area. In fact, flow with healing energy during the entire massage and walk away revitalized! Instead of stopping the massage while you utilize healing techniques, keep slight movement going as you send energy to specific areas. It will give the treatment more continuity.

Distance Healing

At times, we are faced with the desire to help someone who is in another city or state. Since thought is energy, it makes a nice light traveling companion! The process is very similar to regular healing, except that you do it entirely with thought. Take the triple awareness breath, hold the healee in your focus, and begin. You may even scan the person with your thoughts to see what you pick up. Intentionally send healing energy as you hold them in a vision of radiant health. When you've finished, terminate as usual.

On a larger scale, you can also send healing to the earth. Surround it with white light; send healing into the soil, water and air. *Send healing light and love to people everywhere.*

More Ideas For Living In Healing Ways

- Never miss an opportunity for a hearty laugh. Your immune system will be grateful!

- Walk outdoors. As you walk, grab every opportunity to marvel at nature's splendor!

- Breathe! It's natures way of enhancing every cell and getting rid of toxins. Periodically take in a deep breath through your nose...hold it...and then exhale through your mouth.

- Take in the healing rays of the morning sun.

- Meditate.

- Do the Magnificent 7 daily. (You're worth it!)

- Clean your "emotional house" daily. Stay up-to-date with your forgiveness and "I love you's."

- Eat thoughtfully with the idea you are building a healthy body. Choose more and more foods that are in their natural state.

- Drink lots of water, preferably purified water. When you are dining out and you're asked what you'd like to drink, say, "WATER!"

- Have a massage regularly. (You didn't think I'd miss that one, did you?)

- RECEIVE as well as you GIVE. Look for ways to excel in both areas. Continually strive for balance.

- Be aware of other modalities that are health promoting such as acupuncture, acupressure, colonics, reflexology, bio-feedback, guided imagery, etc.

- Learn to make the most of the moment for self-nurturing. In one minute you can unruffle yourself, take some deep breaths, pull in healing energy and drink some water. Imagine what you can do in five or ten minutes!

- Thank your "parts" as you bathe! It goes something like, "Thank you legs, I love you!" "Thank you FEET!" etc. (They're listening!)

- Begin looking more deeply into the eyes of all those you come in contact with to see who's really there (including your own eyes reflecting in the mirror!).

- Be your own best friend!

- Sing or dance until you become one with the music or one with the dance.

- Learn to let the child inside you come out to play. Fly a kite, watch clouds, skip, play hopscotch, sing, dance, fingerpaint, play catch, color, etc.

- Celebrate life daily as you LIVE CONSCIOUSLY IN HEALING WAYS!

Perhaps you've figured out by now that thought is the single most powerful tool you have. Nestled in thought are both your intention and intuition; rather like the gatekeepers to the unlimited...and the profound.

Touching with "intention" provides groundwork for a wonderful "inner journey." More and more you will find yourself intuitively knowing what to do; more and more the specific techniques which have provided "training wheels" will gradually fall away. More and more you will become one with the process, one with the flow. And each time you experience the flow of life force, you have at the same time touched that innermost you...adding an inner harmony that allows you to perceive life in a fresh new way...with a sense of wholeness...a sense of connectedness with all living things. It is a divine moment of listening and blending with all life everywhere. In that moment, you have subtly but surely changed. In that same moment, in a most gentle and special way, *the world has also been touched with intention.* (Hold that thought!)

Suggested Resources
For Working And Living in Healing Ways

Bethard, Betty. *The Dream Book*. Petaluma, CA: Inner Light Foundation, 1995.

Ban Breathnach, Sarah. *Simple Abundance*. New York, New York: Warner Books, Inc., 1995.

Brennan, Barbara. *Hands of Light*. New York, New York: Bantam Books, 1987.

Bruyere, Rosalyn L. *Wheels of Light*. Arcadia, CA: Bon Productions, 1989.

Chiappone, Judie. *Sacred Choices: The gentle art of disarming a disease and reclaiming your Joy!* Winter Springs, Florida: Holistic Reflections, 2000.

Chiappone, Judie. *Sacred Choices for People Undergoing Chemotherapy*. (audio tape) Winter Springs, Florida: Holistic Reflections, 2000.

Chopra, Deepak. *Quantum Healing*. New York: Bantam Books, 1989.

Gordon, Richard. *Your Healing Hands*. Berkeley, CA: Wingbow Press, 1984.

Hay, Louise. *Heal Your Body*. CA: The Hay House, 1988.

Highstein, Max. *The Healing Waterfall*. (audio tape) Upland, CA: 1989.

Krieger, Dolores. *The Therapeutic Touch*. Englewood Cliffs, NJ: Prentice-Hall, Inc., 1979.

Moss, Richard. *The Black Butterfly, An Invitation to Radical Aliveness*. Berkeley, CA: Celestial Arts, 1986.

Northrup, Christiane. *Women's Bodies, Women's Wisdom*. New York, New York: Bantam, 1998.

Siegel, Bernie. *Love, Medicine and Miracles*. New York: Harper and Row, 1986.

Walsch, Neal Donald. *Conversations with God*. Charlottesville, VA: Hampton Roads Publishing Company, 1995.

Williamson, Marianne. *A Return To Love*. New York: Harper Collins, 1989.